The Frith Prescribing Guidelines for People with Intellectual Disability

The Frith Prescribing Guidelines for People with Intellectual Disability

EDITED BY

Professor Sabyasachi Bhaumik, OBE, MBBS, DPM, FRCPsych, Consultant Psychiatrist,

Leicestershire Partnership NHS Trust,
Honorary Chair in Psychiatry, University of Leicester

David Branford, PhD, FRPharmS, FCMHP, Chairman,

English Pharmacy Board, Royal Pharmaceutical Society

Dr Mary Barrett, MBChB, MRCPsych,

Consultant Psychiatrist,
Leicestershire Partnership NHS Trust

Dr Satheesh Kumar Gangadharan, MD, Dip NB, FRCPsych,

Consultant Psychiatrist and Medical Director,
Leicestershire Partnership NHS Trust

THIRD EDITION

WILEY Blackwell

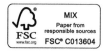

Contents

List of contributors

Regi Alexander
Partnerships in Care, Norfolk & Norwich Medical School
University of East Anglia
Norfolk, UK

Mary Barrett
Leicestershire Partnership NHS Trust
Leicester, UK

Sabyasachi Bhaumik
Leicestershire Partnership NHS Trust
and
Consultant Psychiatrist
Department of Health Sciences, University of Leicester
Leicester, UK

Asit Biswas
Leicestershire Partnership NHS Trust
Leicester, UK

Elspeth Bradley
Surrey Place Centre
and
Department of Psychiatry
University of Toronto
Toronto, Ontario, Canada

David Bramble
Shropshire Community Health NHS Trust
Shrewsbury, UK

David Branford
Chairman
English Pharmacy Board, Royal Pharmaceutical Society
London, UK;
Specialist Pharmacist (retired)

Karen Bretherton
Leicestershire Partnership NHS Trust
Leicester, UK

Nicky Calow
Leicestershire Partnership NHS Trust
Leicester, UK

John Devapriam
Leicestershire Partnership NHS Trust
Leicester, UK

Shweta Gangavati
Leicestershire Partnership NHS Trust
Leicester, UK

Pancho Ghatak
Partnerships in Care
Nottinghamshire, UK

Rohit Gumber
Leicestershire Partnership NHS Trust
Leicester, UK

Avinash Hiremath
Leicestershire Partnership NHS Trust
Leicester, UK

Amala Jovia Maria Jesu
Leicestershire Partnership NHS Trust
Leicester, UK

Sayeed Khan
Leicestershire Partnership NHS Trust
Leicester, UK

Reza Kiani
Leicestershire Partnership NHS Trust
Leicester, UK

Satheesh Kumar Gangadharan
Leicestershire Partnership NHS Trust
Leicester, UK

Dasari Mohan Michael
Humber NHS Foundation Trust
East Riding of Yorkshire, UK

Julia Middleton
Leicestershire Partnership NHS Trust
and
Inclusion Healthcare
Leicester, UK

Helen Miller
National Deaf Service, South West London and St Georges Mental Health NHS Trust
Springfield University Hospital
London, UK

Khalid Nawab
NHS Lanarkshire
Glasgow, UK

Saduf Riaz
NHS Greater Glasgow and Clyde
Glasgow, UK

Nyunt Nyunt Tin
Northamptonshire Healthcare NHS Foundation Trust
Northampton, UK

Jenny Worsfold
Leicestershire Partnership NHS Trust
Leicester, UK

Foreword

Psychiatry of intellectual disability is one of the most complex, stimulating and challenging (in more ways than one) psychiatric specialities. This speciality is an excellent example of the closest and most complex interactions between physical and psychiatric symptoms. This interaction can lead to both diagnostic and management challenges. Working with people with intellectual disabilities across the lifespan also raises serious challenges in getting the medical interventions right in combination with psychological and social interventions.

Knowing the right medication is one task, but getting the doses right is a bigger challenge for clinicians working in the field. The complex interaction between physical and mental health and the relationship between intellectual disability and psychiatric illnesses mean that special care must be taken while prescribing and also looking out for side effects.

This third edition (the first edition was published nearly a decade ago) is to be hugely welcomed. Its chapters cover a whole range of psychiatric conditions. Impressively, they also include gender-related illnesses, which are too often ignored.

The editors have taken tremendous amount of effort to get the medication and doses right, making sure that the patients get the prescribed right doses of right medications and based on current evidence the patients get the best treatment they need and deserve. The book is now in its third edition, which in itself speaks high volumes for its quality and the need for such a book.

My congratulations to the editors for creating an excellent volume and for their continuing efforts and energy in ensuring that patients with intellectual disability and mental disorders get the most suitable and appropriate treatments.

Dinesh Bhugra, CBE, MA, MSc, MBBS, FRCP, FRCPE, FRCPsych, FFPH, MPhil, PhD
Professor of Mental Health and Cultural Diversity
Institute of Psychiatry (King's College London)
President-Elect World Psychiatric Association 2014–2017

Preface

This is the third edition of the *Frith Prescribing Guidelines* and remains the only prescribing guideline in the UK specifically targeted at people with intellectual disability, to the best of our knowledge. Since the first edition in 2005, the scientific evidence base has gradually gathered in strength; the second edition in 2008 drew together that evidence base while still retaining consensus opinion for those areas where the science remained lacking. This third edition builds on the previous ones but also seeks to acknowledge the clinical complexity perpetually encountered in the psychiatry of intellectual disability. For the third edition, the editors therefore decided to include case examples, designed to both illustrate the practical application of that evidence base and also draw out some of the clinical complexities for further discussion and consideration by the reader. The answers to the Discussion Case Studies can be found in Chapter 20. We hope that this format proves useful and would welcome feedback on this, and indeed any other aspects of the book, from readers to inform future editions.

Sabyasachi Bhaumik, David Branford, Mary Barrett
and Satheesh Kumar Gangadharan

Acknowledgements

The editors would like to thank all those who have given their time and expertise to help produce this third edition of the *Frith Prescribing Guidelines*.

Particular mention must go to Professor Dinesh Bhugra, MA, MSc, MBBS, FRCP, FRCPE, FRCPsych, FFPH, MPhil, PhD, Professor of Mental Health and Cultural Diversity, Institute of Psychiatry (King's College London) CBE, for kindly providing the Foreword and also to Dr Elspeth Bradley, PhD, FRCPC, FRCPsych, Psychiatrist-in-Chief Surrey Place Centre, Associate Professor, Department of Psychiatry, University of Toronto, Canada, for her advice and support and for providing an international perspective.

The principal contributors to each chapter of the third edition are listed here. Without them, this book could not have been produced. The editors would also like to thank many of our colleagues nationally for helping us develop these guidelines through their advice and suggestions.

1	Intellectual disability	David Branford and Sabyasachi Bhaumik
2	Prescribing practice	David Branford and Sabyasachi Bhaumik
3	Physical and health monitoring	David Branford and Sabyasachi Bhaumik
4	Epilepsy	Reza Kiani and David Branford
5	Dementia in people with intellectual disability	Satheesh Kumar Gangadharan and Amala Jovia Maria Jesu
6	Eating and drinking difficulties	Jenny Worsfold, Nicky Calow and David Branford
7	Sleep disorders	Reza Kiani and David Bramble
8	Women's Health issues	Nyunt Nyunt Tin and Julia Middleton
9	Sexual Disorders	John Devapriam, Pancho Ghatak, Sabyasachi Bhaumik, David Branford, Mary Barrett and Sayeed Khan
10	Autism spectrum disorders	Mary Barrett and Elspeth Bradley
11	ADHD	Karen Bretherton
12	Aggressive behaviour	David Branford and Sabyasachi Bhaumik
13	Self-injurious behaviour	Asit Biswas and Sabyasachi Bhaumik
14	Anxiety disorders	Avinash Hiremath, Sabyasachi Bhaumik and Khalid Nawab
15	Depression	Avinash Hiremath, Shweta Gangavati, Rohit Gumber and Mary Barrett
16	Bipolar affective disorder	Desari Mohan Michael, David Branford and Mary Barrett

17	Schizophrenia	Avinash Hiremath, Amala Jovia Maria Jesu, Rohit Gumber and Saduf Riaz
18	Alcohol use disorders	Helen Miller
19	Personality disorders	Regi Alexander and Sabyasachi Bhaumik

The editors would also like to thank all the contributors to the previous editions, on which this edition has been built. Particular mention and thanks go to Dr Agnes Hauck, Dr Sanyogita Nadkarni, Dr Joanna M Watson, Dr Lammata Bala Raju, Dr Tim Betts, Professor Shoumitro Deb, Dr Sisir Majumdar, Dr Amitava Das Gupta, Ms Christine Pacitti, Ms Gaynor Ward, Ms Rachel Walsh and Ms Alison MacKinnon.

CHAPTER 1

Intellectual Disability

David Branford[1] & Sabyasachi Bhaumik[2,3]

[1]English Pharmacy Board, Royal Pharmaceutical Society, London, UK
[2]Leicestershire Partnership NHS Trust, Leicester, UK
[3]Department of Health Sciences, University of Leicester, Leicester, UK

> Whatever term is chosen for this condition, it eventually becomes perceived as an insult.
>
> *Wikipedia*

Throughout time, many terms have been used to describe the condition now we currently call intellectual disability (ID). Wikipedia describes the evolution of these many terms, including mental retardation (United States) and mental handicap (United Kingdom) and how each, in turn, becomes incorporated into normal language in a derogatory way.

There is a general consensus on the concept of ID. It requires the presence of three criteria based on the definition derived after extensive consultation in the United States (Luckasson et al., 1992). These criteria have been carried forwards in DSM-5.

The American Psychiatric Association (APA) diagnostic criteria for ID (DSM-5 criteria) are as follows:

1. Deficits in general mental abilities.
2. Impairment in adaptive functioning for individual's age and sociocultural background, which may include communication, social skills, person independence and school or work functioning.
3. All symptoms must have an onset during the developmental period.

The condition may be subcategorised according to severity based on adaptive functioning as mild, moderate and severe.

Significant intellectual impairment is usually defined as an intelligence quotient (IQ) more than 2 standard deviations below the general population mean (originally fixed at 100). This is an IQ below 70 on recognised IQ tests. Two per cent of the population have an IQ below this level. Significant deficits in social

---

The Frith Prescribing Guidelines for People with Intellectual Disability, Third Edition.
Edited by Sabyasachi Bhaumik, David Branford, Mary Barrett and Satheesh Kumar Gangadharan.
© 2015 John Wiley & Sons, Ltd. Published 2015 by John Wiley & Sons, Ltd.

functioning are commonly measured using well-known scales such as the Vineland Adaptive Behaviour Scales (VABS) or the Adaptive Behaviour Assessment System (ABAS II). These assess communication, daily living skills and socialisation; the VABS also assesses motor skills.

The term 'ID' is used in this text synonymously with learning disability (the common terminology currently used in clinical practice in the United Kingdom), mental retardation (used in ICD-10 and DSM-IV) and mental handicap (used in the United Kingdom until 1994). A decision to use ID was based upon this being currently the most widely recognised and acceptable term for an international readership.

The 11th revision of ICD is underway and the WHO has established several working groups to contribute to the beta phase of the 11th revision. At this stage, the proposal is for changing the name of the disorder from 'mental retardation' to 'disorders of intellectual development'.

The term 'learning difficulty', first proposed by the Warnock Committee, is a much broader category than ID. This is the term used in the UK educational system. Learning difficulties include speech and language impairments; learning problems arising from sensory impairments, physical disabilities, medical problems or behaviour difficulties; and specific learning problems such as dyslexia. ID is associated with global impairment of intellectual and adaptive functioning and is assessed using intellectual criteria; learning difficulty is assessed by educational criteria. The measures for the latter are mostly proxy measures of learning achievement (rather than the learning process itself) such as memory recall, reading, number and problem solving. It is estimated that about one in five children has a learning difficulty at some time during the course of life, and one in six children has a learning difficulty at any one time. These guidelines refer to adults with ID and learning difficulties will not be considered further.

Prevalence

The prevalence of ID depends on the cut-off point used for the definition of ID (Table 1.1) and the methodology used to measure it. Studies that have screened whole populations tend to find a higher prevalence (around 6 per 1000 population) than those that include only those known to services, the administrative prevalence. It is estimated that the prevalence is increasing at a rate of 1% a year.

Table 1.1 Administrative prevalence of ID in the UK.

Severity of ID	IQ	Prevalence per 1000 population
Mild	50–69	30
Moderate	35–49	}
Severe	20–34	} 3
Profound	<20	0.5

Aetiology

Biological, environmental and social factors may contribute to the development of ID. A large number of different aetiological processes may be involved; these are usually complex and often not completely understood. Biological factors are present in about 67–75% of people with ID, the majority operating before birth (Table 1.2). The two most common genetic causes are Down syndrome and Fragile X syndrome. In a third of people with ID, no primary diagnosis can be made.

Table 1.2 Biological factors that may cause ID.

Period of origin	Nature of disorder	Common examples
Prenatal period	**Genetic disorders**	
	Chromosome aberrations	Down syndrome (trisomy 21)
	Single gene mutations	Tuberous sclerosis,
	Microdeletions	phenylketonuria,
		mucopolysaccharidoses, fragile X
		syndrome
		Prader–Willi syndrome, Williams
		syndrome
	Congenital malformations	
	Central nervous system malformations	Neural tube defects
	Multiple malformation syndromes	Cornelia de Lange syndrome
	Exposure	
	Maternal infections	Congenital rubella, HIV
	Teratogens	Foetal alcohol syndrome
	Toxaemia, placental insufficiency	Prematurity
	Severe malnutrition	Intra-uterine growth retardation
	Trauma	Physical injury
	Iatrogenic	Radiation, medications
Perinatal period	Infections	TORCH infections: toxoplasmosis,
	Delivery	hepatitis B, syphilis, herpes zoster,
	Other causes	rubella, cytomegalovirus, herpes
		simplex
		Anoxic brain damage
		Hyperbilirubinaemia
Postnatal period	Infections	Encephalitis
	Metabolic	Hypoglycaemia
	Endocrine	Hypothyroidism (cretinism)
	Cerebrovascular	Thrombo-embolic phenomena
	Toxins	Lead poisoning
	Trauma	Head injury
	Neoplasms	Meningioma, craniopharyngioma
	Psychosocial factors	Understimulation
Any	Untraceable or unknown	

How common are health needs in people with ID?

- People with ID have significantly more health problems than the general population.
- People with ID have a shorter life expectancy and increased risk of early death when compared to the general population.
- All-cause mortality rates among people with moderate to severe ID are three times higher than in the general population, with mortality being particularly high for young adults, women and people with Down syndrome.
- The prevalence of psychiatric disorders is 36% among children with ID, compared to 8% among children without ID.
- The prevalence of psychiatric disorders is also significantly higher among adults with ID when compared to general population rates.
- Around 50% of adults have a major psychiatric or behaviour problem requiring specialist help.
- Twenty-five per cent of adults with ID have active epilepsy, at least 33% have a sensory impairment, and around 40% have associated major physical disabilities of mobility and incontinence.
- Fifty to ninety per cent of people with ID have communication difficulties; a lack of supported communication may compound their problems in receiving the healthcare that they need.

The substantial health needs of this population are often overlooked and unmet, something that has been highlighted by reports including 'Treat Me Right!' (MENCAP), 'Death by Indifference' (MENCAP) and 'Equal Treatment: Closing the Gap' (DRC). Sometimes, this reaches the level of national outrage, as with the mistreatment of people with ID at the inpatient assessment facility Winterbourne View, near Bristol in the United Kingdom, which was shut down and where a number of staff were prosecuted.

How do psychiatric and behavioural problems present in ID?

Both the diagnosis and treatment of psychiatric and behavioural problems in people with ID may need a different approach from that in the general population. Although there are guidelines to assist practitioners in prescribing medications for mental health problems in the wider population, the Frith Guidelines are the first to address the specific issues relating to the pharmacological treatment of mental health and other problems in adults with ID.

Psychiatric and behaviour problems often present differently in adults with ID from the presentation commonly seen in the general population. The symptoms may be mistakenly attributed to the ID itself, a phenomenon known as diagnostic overshadowing. In addition, symptoms of an underlying physical condition or a reaction to environmental changes may mask those of an additional psychiatric disturbance. Difficulties in diagnosis may be further compounded by the communication difficulties experienced by people with ID. Furthermore, for many conditions, there is a lack of suitable diagnostic criteria or instruments.

What is the evidence base for medication treatment in ID?

In the psychiatry of ID, the evidence base for the use of psychotropic medications is extremely limited. There are few well-designed randomised controlled trials (RCTs). Adults with ID frequently have additional health problems that preclude them from being recruited into studies. The National Institute for Health and Care Excellence (NICE) has not yet produced guidelines specifically for the ID population. A guideline produced by Deb et al. (2006) in collaboration with MENCAP and the Royal College of Psychiatrists is limited to the medication management of behaviour problems. Further guidelines are awaited following the national response to Winterbourne View.

Consequent to the lack of evidence, a wide range of psychotropic medications are currently used outside their licensed indications to manage challenging behaviours, which may or may not be associated with an underlying mental health problem. For example, 23% of the ID population are prescribed antipsychotics for behavioural disturbances. The reasons for this are many, including:

- Pressure from professionals/carers for immediate resolution of a problem
- Limited resources available for changing the environment
- Lack of appropriately trained staff in private residential homes
- Shortfall of psychiatrists
- Lack of input from clinical psychologists, specialist, clinical pharmacists and speech therapists

Even with the use of optimum resources and good professional input, some behaviour problems remain unchanged, causing serious risk to the person and others. In some cases, the use of psychotropic medications brings welcome relief to all concerned; for example, using low-dose risperidone in those with an autism spectrum disorder may reduce stereotypies and disturbed behaviour. In some, medications can work to reduce elevated arousal levels, allowing the person to engage in other therapeutic approaches. Nevertheless, clinicians who use psychotropic medications outside their licensed indications feel vulnerable and open to criticism for 'unethical practice', and strong views exist about 'chemical straitjacketing' for behaviour disorders in the absence of adequate resources.

Pharmacokinetic and pharmacodynamic issues in ID

Although there is evidence that people with ID may handle medications differently from the general population, this is by no means proven. Within the ID population, there is greater variation in the physical stature and physiological functioning than in the wider population. Such factors may result in different electrolyte and blood values, different volumes of distribution and different renal and hepatic capacity. These, in turn, may affect the pharmacokinetics and efficacy of a medication. The nature of the damage in the brain or changes in the brain structure that have given rise to the ID may result in

- altered sensitivities to a medication
- changed effects of the medication
- difficulties in determining the optimum dose.

There is anecdotal evidence that people with ID experience more adverse medication reactions than the general population, but again this remains unproven. Studies show inconclusive results, possibly because of communication problems and reporting difficulties. There has been widespread concern in the past about the use of typical antipsychotics because of their propensity to cause the long-term irreversible movement disorder called tardive dyskinesia. However, studies of the prevalence of tardive dyskinesia following long-term use of antipsychotics show mixed results. Similarly now there are now concerns regarding the newer atypical antipsychotics and their association with the side effects of weight gain, diabetes and the metabolic syndrome. Again it is also unclear whether people with ID are at greater risk (see Chapter 2).

Also there are specific medications that present a greater benefit or hazard to adults with ID than adults in the general population, for example, anticholinergics for dribbling, eye drops, laxatives or hormone-replacement therapy. Nevertheless, multiple health problems and consequent multiple medication use put persons with ID at increased risk of adverse medication reactions and medication interactions.

Why this guideline?

A number of guidelines concerning general principles for the use of psychotropic medications have been published. These include the *International Consensus Handbook* (United States), *The Expert Consensus Guideline for the Treatment of Psychiatric and Behavioural Problems in Mental Retardation* (United States) and guidelines for using medication to manage behavioural problems (United Kingdom). These guidelines are reviewed in Chapter 2.

The Frith Guidelines have been written in response to the clinical challenges faced by clinicians. Their purpose is to allow standardised practice across ID, moving away from idiosyncratic prescribing towards a consensus approach based on both evidence and expert opinion. However, every person referred to ID services is unique; therefore, there may be a considerable variation in the clinical approaches used. Hence, this book has been produced as a guideline only, *not* as a protocol.

The guidelines were written after a thorough examination of the current evidence base, followed by a series of peer reviews with clinicians from national clinical centres. The peer group included representatives from health districts in London and South–East Thames; the West Midlands and the Trent Region; Partnerships in

Care, Norfolk; the Academic Centre of the University of Birmingham; and the Neurology Services of the West Midlands. The current NICE guidelines in relevant areas have been incorporated where possible, including those for dementia, bipolar affective disorder and schizophrenia, with relevant modifications for those with ID.

Although the guidelines will be revised periodically, with the rapid growth and development of pharmacology and the continuing publication of NICE guidelines, readers are advised to keep abreast of recent developments and to modify the guidelines accordingly between publications. These guidelines should not be used in isolation but seen as part of a holistic package of care that includes non-pharmacological approaches such as psychological input, community support, dealing with underlying physical problems and addressing environmental and social issues pertinent to the person. The core of real clinical improvement lies in a thorough understanding of the issues involved, empathy and rapport with patients and carers and a thorough clinical assessment. It is these parameters that determine the success or failure of any treatment rather than a strict adherence to protocols or guidelines.

Key issues in working with people with ID

Communication

Difficulties in communication may make it more difficult for the clinician to ascertain the nature and extent of any benefits and side effects of prescribing a medication for a patient with ID. When a patient is living independently, it is crucial to communicate the need to take the medicine and the instructions for taking it. Simple written or pictorial instructions may help understanding and compliance. It may be prudent to ensure that support is in place to monitor that the medication is taken and, if required, to monitor blood levels of the medication. When a patient is being cared for by others, it is important that the carers understand the purpose of the medicine, how it should be given and what parameters need to be monitored. When eliciting and giving information about epilepsy and other complex phenomena, clear simple language should be used rather than medical terms.

Consent

Whenever possible, express consent should be obtained from the patient before beginning treatment. This is in accordance with General Medical Council (GMC) guidance. Express consent usually means consent that is expressed orally or in writing; however, where a person cannot speak or write, other forms of communication may be sufficient.

For a person's consent to be legally valid and professionally acceptable, they must be:
• Capable of taking that particular decision (competent)
• Acting voluntarily

- Provided with enough information (in a form that he/she can understand) to enable him/her to make the decision

For adults with ID, this is often a process over time rather than a 'one-off' effort. The Mental Capacity Act makes it clear that one should assume that any person *has* the capacity to give consent until evidence to the contrary is shown. A person cannot be considered to lack capacity until reasonable measures are taken to enhance his/her decision-making ability. In a person with ID, particular attention should be paid to:

- The mode of communication (particularly the use of communication aids)
- The environment in which information is provided
- The person's familiarity to whoever provides the information
- The pace at which the information is provided

Broadly, incapacity means that a person is unable, by the reason of impaired mental ability, to make a decision for him-/herself on the matter in question or to communicate that decision. No one can give consent on behalf of an adult who lacks capacity. The assessment of an adult patient's capacity to make a decision about his/her own medical treatment is a matter of clinical judgement guided by the Mental Capacity Act. It is the personal responsibility of any professional proposing to treat a patient to judge whether the patient has the capacity to give valid consent. The clinician has a duty to give the patient an account in simple terms of the nature of the treatment, benefits versus risks of the proposed treatment and the main alternative options.

Demonstrating a person's capacity

A person should be able to:
- Understand in simple language what the medical treatment is, its purpose and nature and why it is being proposed
- Understand its principal benefits, risks and options
- Understand in broad terms what will be the consequences of not receiving the proposed treatment
- Retain the information for long enough to make an effective decision
- Weigh that information in the balance and arrive at a free choice
- Communicate their decision

NB: All assessments of a patient's capacity should be fully recorded in their medical notes.

There are occasions when some forms of medical treatment are lawful in the absence of the patient's consent. The concept of necessity permits clinicians to provide treatment without obtaining consent if:

1 There is a necessity to act when it is not practicable to communicate with the assisted person.

2 The action taken is such that a reasonable person would take, given all the circumstances, acting in the best interests of the person who is being assisted.

Not only may a clinician give treatment to an incapacitated patient when it is clearly in that person's best interests, but it is also a common law duty to do so.

In day-to-day clinical practice, decisions regarding treatments are taken for adults who lack capacity using best interest principles. There is a clear guidance for formulating a best interest decision in the Mental Capacity Act. Key principles are:

• The person remains at the centre of the decision-making process and participates as much as they are able.
• Parents, carers and other people close to the patient need to be consulted for information about the patient's preferences, choices and best interests.
• Consideration needs to be given to the least restrictive option for the patient's rights and freedom.
• For decisions regarding serious medical treatment or a change in accommodation when a person is classed as 'unbefriended' (has no one to speak for them apart from professionals/paid carers), then involvement of an independent mental capacity advocate (IMCA) is to be obtained.
• Intervention from the newly established Court of Protection could be sought for treatment decisions that are more serious or contentious.

A detailed discussion of capacity to consent is beyond the scope of these guidelines; we recommend the use of Mental Capacity Act and its associated Code of Practice.

The principles and procedures for the detention of a person for assessment or treatment or other purposes under the provisions of the Mental Health Act 1983 are the same as for the general population. Further details are beyond the scope of this guideline.

References

Deb S, Clarke D, Unwin G (2006) *Using medication to manage behaviour problems among adults with a learning disability: quick reference guide (QRG)*. London: University of Birmingham, MENCAP, The Royal College of Psychiatrists.

Luckasson R, Coulter DL, Polloway EA, et al. (1992) *Mental retardation: definition, classification, and systems of supports* (9th ed.). Washington, DC: American Association on Mental Retardation.

Further reading

American Psychiatric Association (2013) *Diagnostic and statistical manual of mental disorders* (5th ed.). Arlington, VA: American Psychiatric Publishing.

Cooper SA, Smiley E, Morrison J, Williamson A, Allan L (2007) Mental ill-health in adults with intellectual disabilities: prevalence and associated factors. *British Journal of Psychiatry* 190:27–35.

Department for Constitutional Affairs (DCA) (2007) Mental Capacity Act 2005, Code of Practice. London: DCA, The Stationery Office. http://www.direct.gov.uk/prod_consum_dg/groups/dg_digitalassets/@dg/@en/@disabled/documents/digitalasset/dg_186484.pdf (accessed 6 January 2015).

Department of Health (2009) *Reference guide to consent for examination or treatment* (2nd ed.). London: Crown. www.dh.gov.uk/publications (accessed 6 January 2015).

Department of Health (2012) DH Winterbourne view review. Concordat: programme of action. https://www.gov.uk/government/uploads/system/uploads/attachment_data/file/213217/Concordat.pdf (accessed 6 January 2015).

Department of Health, Social Services and Public Safety, Northern Ireland (2003) Seeking consent: working with people with learning disabilities. http://www.dhsspsni.gov.uk/consent-guidepart4.pdf (accessed 6 January 2015).

Foundation for People with Learning Disabilities (n.d.) Learning disability a–z. http://www.learningdisabilities.org.uk/help-information/learning-disability-a-z (accessed 6 January 2015).

General Medical Council (n.d.) Consent guidance: patients and doctors making decisions together. http://www.gmc-uk.org/guidance/ethical_guidance/consent_guidance_index.asp (accessed 6 January 2015).

McGrother CW, Thorp CF, Taub N, Machado O (2001) Prevalence, disability and need in adults with severe learning disability. *Tizard Learning Disability Review* 6:4–13.

MENCAP (2007) *Death by indifference.* London: MENCAP.

Office of the Public Guardian. Mental Capacity Act: making decisions. http://www.justice.gov.uk/protecting-the-vulnerable/mental-capacity-act (accessed 6 January 2015).

Royal College of Nursing (2013) Making it work. Shared decision-making and people with learning disabilities. RCN Policy and International Department, RCN Nursing Department, Policy briefing 41/12. http://www.rcn.org.uk/__data/assets/pdf_file/0003/526503/41.12_Making_it_work_Shared_decision-making_and_people_with_learning_disabilities.pdf (accessed 6 January 2015).

Tyrer F, McGrother C (2009) Cause-specific mortality and death certificate reporting in adults with moderate to profound intellectual disabilities. *Journal of Intellectual Disability Research* 53:898–904.

CHAPTER 2

Prescribing Practice

David Branford[1] & Sabyasachi Bhaumik[2,3]

[1]*English Pharmacy Board, Royal Pharmaceutical Society, London, UK*
[2]*Leicestershire Partnership NHS Trust, Leicester, UK*
[3]*Department of Health Sciences, University of Leicester, Leicester, UK*

New medicines, and new methods of cures, always work miracles for a while.

William Heberden, 1710–1801

Definition

Psychotropic medications are commonly prescribed for people with intellectual disability (ID) for the treatment of psychiatric and behavioural problems. For the purposes of this chapter, any medication or substance used to treat, improve or stabilise mood, mental state or behaviour is regarded as a psychotropic medication. This includes sedatives, antipsychotics, anxiolytics, stimulants, antidepressants, hypnotics and other medications not normally regarded as psychotropic (e.g. antiepileptic drugs) when used to improve mood or behaviour. It also includes herbal or nutritional substances when used to improve mood or behaviour.

Prevalence

Surveys undertaken in a wide range of countries indicate that 30–40% of patients with ID living in institutional care and 10–20% of those living in community settings receive psychotropic medication. Antipsychotics have been in the past, and still are, the main group used; however, other medications such as antiepileptics for mood stabilisation and antidepressants have become more widely prescribed in recent years.

The Frith Prescribing Guidelines for People with Intellectual Disability, Third Edition.
Edited by Sabyasachi Bhaumik, David Branford, Mary Barrett and Satheesh Kumar Gangadharan.

Categories of psychotropic medication use

Psychotropic medication used in ID generally falls into the following categories:
- Treatment of mental illness (MI), for example, schizophrenia and affective disorders
- Management of challenging behaviours not caused by MI that impact adversely on the person with ID or others
- Management of behaviours associated with autism spectrum disorders that interfere with daily functioning, such as stereotypical repetitive behaviours
- Rapid tranquillisation for the short-term control of violent and aggressive behaviour
- Stimulants for the management of attention deficit
- Acetylcholinesterase inhibitors and other medications to delay the cognitive decline and other impacts of dementia
- Hypnotics for the management of sleep

Are psychotropic medications overprescribed for people with ID?

Evidence from many surveys suggests that, particularly in the management of challenging behaviours, psychotropic medications – and in particular antipsychotic drugs – are overprescribed. During the many enquiries associated with the Winterbourne scandal in the UK, there also arose concerns that, in addition to antipsychotic drugs, other groups of psychotropic medication were being widely used with little evidence to support their use. These included antidepressants, mood stabilisers and benzodiazepines.

Polypharmacy

Polypharmacy has many definitions, ranging from more than one medication from the same class, multiple medications prescribed for the same problem, multiple medications and even medications that are unnecessary. In view of this for the purposes of clarity, the authors of the Frith Guidelines have agreed the following definitions:
- Polypharmacy is the use of more than one medication from the same class, for example, antipsychotic polypharmacy is the prescribing of more than one antipsychotic and antidepressant polypharmacy is the prescribing of more than one antidepressant.

Polypharmacy can be both regular and potential:
- Regular polypharmacy is when the person receives more than one medication from the same class as a part of their regular medication.
- Potential polypharmacy is when the person is prescribed in addition to a regular medication from the same class an as-required medication from the same class.

Antiepileptic polypharmacy, as described previously, is common in people with ID for the treatment of epilepsy. This has been exacerbated in recent years by the introduction of many new antiepileptics. It is usual for these new antiepileptics to be introduced as an add-on therapy and for refractory epilepsy. Many people with ID and epilepsy remain refractory to treatment, and antiepileptic polypharmacy is common.

There are similar concerns with the treatment of challenging behaviours. Although antipsychotic prescribing is a widespread issue in the management of challenging behaviours in ID, antipsychotic polypharmacy is not. However, the prescribing of CNS-active medications from a variety of different categories has become a concern. Some authors have used the term polytherapy to describe receiving many medicines for many conditions; however, in order to achieve clarity, we will use the term CNS polytherapy to describe multiple CNS-active medication use.

In recent years, it has become common for people with ID to be prescribed medication from a wide variety of sources and for a wide variety of medications to be prescribed as a part of normal management of many illnesses and problems. For example, within diabetes care or hypertension, it is not unusual to see the prescribing of three or more medications. Many authors also use the term polypharmacy to describe such multiple medication therapy.

Many of the problems associated with ID, such as epilepsy, challenging behaviours, physical problems or MI, remain a constant feature throughout the person's life. These problems, although helped by medication, commonly remain partially refractory to treatment, and ever-increasing numbers and changes of medication remain a feature of prescribing. Evidence from many studies demonstrates that regular comprehensive medication review involving medical staff, pharmacists and carers results in significant reduction in the prescribing of all types of medication. However, there is also evidence to suggest that:

• Illnesses go unrecognised (particularly those associated with old age).
• People with ID may not access general health-care services that are available to the general population.

Do people with ID handle medication differently from the general population?

For many people with ID, the cause of their disabilities may be damage to the brain. The nature of the damage to brain structures may result in altered sensitivity to medication, changed medication effects and difficulties in determining dose. In addition, aspects of the physical stature and other parameters may result in a different volume of distribution, different electrolyte and blood values and different renal and hepatic capacity. Within the wide range of people encompassed by the term ID, there may be people for whom none of these factors are relevant – the way they deal with medication is the same as the general population. However, for others, the medication may lead to acute or chronic responses of an unexpected nature.

Are people with ID at greater risk of adverse reactions to medication?

This remains unclear. How adverse reactions to medication present in the general population is varied. One could predict that given the physical and structural issues associated with ID, the prevalence of adverse reactions would be greater; however, there is only anecdotal evidence that this is the case. Even studies of side effects such as tardive dyskinesia, hyperprolactinaemia and the metabolic syndrome have produced mixed prevalence results. See below.

> This study compared 138 antipsychotic-treated and 64 antipsychotic-naive participants with ID in one UK National Health Service Trust.
>
> It concluded that antipsychotics, on average, did not increase metabolic risk, although the existence of a susceptible subgroup at risk of diabetes could not be excluded.
>
> Some antipsychotics induced hyperprolactinaemia and hypogonadism, requiring active management. Their findings did suggest that antipsychotics at the low doses routinely prescribed for people with ID are generally safe in relation to metabolic adverse effects, even if efficacy remains poorly defined.
>
> Source: Frighi et al. (2011). © *British Journal of Psychiatry*.

How does communication impact on medication use?

Lack of or limited level of communication skills of people with ID may result in difficulties in diagnosis, difficulties in interpreting the change that has resulted from medication use and difficulties in ascertaining the extent of the side effects. If a person self-cares, communicating the need to take medication and when/how to take it may also present a problem.

The evidence base to support the use of psychotropic medication in ID

As highlighted in Chapter 1, the evidence base to support the use of psychotropic medication in ID remains weak. Most guidelines are based on consensus (as is the Frith Guidelines). The following is information relating to other consensus guidelines. None of the guidelines present recommendations relating to particular medication; however, each provides a template for safer practice.

How effectively are medications for people with ID reviewed?

Whether people with ID are at greater risk of receiving unnecessary or excessive medication remains the subject of many audits and studies. There is no current consensus on whether there is a need to introduce greater scrutiny and oversight for this very vulnerable group or to what extent specialist oversight is required. In Canada, there is no requirement for physicians prescribing these medications to have training in the care of people with ID. Services for people with ID and behaviour problems in Canada were reported by Bradley and Cheetham (2010) to be more crisis reactive than those in the UK.

Two audits below undertaken in the UK of services involving specialists suggest there is not a problem with the indications for the medication, but there may be a problem with the review of physical and metabolic side effects. This would support the need for input of specialists.

> Griffiths et al. collected data from all 178 patients with ID.
> Demographics, severity of ID, co-morbid diagnoses and details of any antipsychotic drug use were collected.
> The main standards of prescribing that were measured included indication of antipsychotic prescribing, documented review of medications, documentation of side effects and documentation of physical health parameters including weight, blood pressure, blood glucose and lipids.
> A third of the sample population was being treated with antipsychotics for behaviour problems.
> The study also shows that there was lack of documentation of physical health and side effect monitoring. It highlights that there should be regular monitoring of physical and side effects with careful documentation.
> Source: Griffiths et al. (2012). © Emerald Group Publishing Ltd.

> Paton et al. through the Prescribing Observatory for Mental Health (POMH–UK) collected a sample comprising 2319 patients with ID from 39 services in the UK that were studied.
> The conclusion was that most prescriptions for antipsychotics in people with ID were consistent with the evidence base and that the overall quality of prescribing practice, a measure against recognised standards, was good although in some patients side effects monitoring was less satisfactory.
> Source: Paton et al. (2011). © Wiley.

How do children with ID compare with adults?

Unwin and Deb (2011) undertook a systematic review of antipsychotic drug use in children with ID. They found the use of medication to manage problem behaviours is widespread, but robust evidence to support their use seemed to be lacking. Their review was of the research evidence into the efficacy of atypical antipsychotic medication in managing problem behaviour in children with ID and borderline intelligence. The review was conducted for placebo-controlled randomised double-blind trials. This included studies ($N=6$) that showed that risperidone was significantly more effective than placebo in managing problem behaviours; however, most studies highlighted adverse events, primarily somnolence and weight gain.

Key guidelines

In 1995, a guideline for the use of psychotropic medication was developed in the USA following an international consensus conference on psychopharmacology. Its summary document proposed 'The 10 dos – 4 don'ts principle' that was later published in 1998 by Kalachnik et al. Although this is now quite old and the medications mentioned have been largely superseded by newer versions, the general advice remains as relevant now as it was in 1998.

Ten dos:
1 Treat any behaviour drug as a psychotropic drug.
2 Use within a coordinated care plan.
3 Base treatment on a diagnosis or specific hypothesis.
4 Obtain written consent.
5 Track efficacy by defining index behaviours.
6 Monitor side effects using rating instruments.
7 Monitor for tardive dyskinesia (NB: this could now be added to by 'monitor for metabolic syndrome').
8 Review systematically and regularly.
9 Strive for lowest optimal effective dose.
10 Monitor use by peer or quality review.

Four don'ts:
1 Don't use psychotropic drugs excessively for convenience or as a substitute for meaningful activity.
2 Avoid frequent drug and dose changes.
3 Avoid intraclass polypharmacy.
4 Minimise:
  • Long-term p.r.n. orders ('pro re nata' or 'as needed')
  • Long-acting sedative/hypnotics
  • Long-term hypnotics or anxiolytics
  • High antipsychotic doses
  • Long-term anticholinergics

In 2000, the *American Journal on Mental Retardation* published an expert consensus guideline for the treatment of psychiatric and behavioural problems in ID (Rush and Frances, 2000). The guideline was based on surveys of 48 experts on psychosocial treatments and 45 experts on treatment with medication. In addition to the above, they recommended that:

A Psychotropic medication use should be based on a psychiatric diagnosis or a specific behavioural–pharmacological hypothesis. This results from a diagnostic and functional assessment that addresses the following:
  • Medical pathology
  • Psychosocial and environmental conditions
  • Health status

- Current medication
- Presence of psychiatric condition
- History, previous interventions and results
- Functional analysis of behaviour

B When determining adequate duration of a medication trial before considering switch to other medication, they advocated:
- Antipsychotics, 3–8 weeks
- Mood stabilisers, 1–3 weeks
- Antidepressants, 6–8 weeks (NB: some studies would suggest that 12 weeks may be needed for older patients)

C Dosing strategies:
- Start low and go slow – use lower initial doses and increase more slowly than in the general population.
- Use same or lower maintenance maximum doses as in general population.
- Periodically consider gradual dose reduction.
- Reduce doses at the same rate or slower than in the general population.

In 2006, Deb et al. developed a quick reference guide 'Using medication to manage behaviour problems among adults with learning disabilities'. This used both expert surveys and critical evaluation of available literature to achieve a consensus. Their guide, in addition to issues raised earlier, identified a wide range of other issues associated with the prescribing of psychotropic medication:

- Background assessment of the behaviours/problems:
  - Ensure an assessment has been conducted and recorded before initiating treatment.
  - Ensure an appropriate formulation is carried out and a treatment plan drawn up, prior to instigating any interventions.
- Physical examinations and investigations:
  - Ensure that appropriate physical examinations and investigations have been carried out.
- Discussions with service users or their family or carers:
  - Assess the person's capacity to consent to treatment.
  - Discuss the formulation and treatment plan with the person and/or their family or carers.
- Issues relating to the use of unlicensed medication:
  - Clarify to the person and/or their family or carers if the medication is prescribed outside their licensed indication.
- Information sharing and provision of written information:
  - Discuss the formulation and treatment plan with other relevant professionals.
  - Provide the person and/or their family or carers with a written treatment plan.
- Follow-up assessments:
  - Agree the method and timing of assessing treatment outcome along with a follow-up date for review of treatment progress.

Recent guidance from the Royal College of Psychiatrists (UK)

Following the 2009 international guidance, the Royal College of Psychiatrists (RCPsych) UK produced guidance with an audit tool. Their general principles for prescribing psychotropic medications are as below.

Anyone prescribing medication to manage problem behaviours in adults with ID should keep the following good practice points in mind:

- Medication should be used only in the best interests of the person.
- All non-medication management options should be considered, and medication should be seen as necessary under the circumstances or alongside non-medication management.
- If possible, evidence to show that the medication is cost-effective should be taken into account.
- Information about which medications worked before and which did not should be noted.
- If medication used previously produced unacceptable adverse effects, the details should be noted.
- The effect of availability or non-availability of certain services and therapies on the treatment plan should be taken into account.
- Relevant local and national protocols and guidelines should be followed.

References

Bradley E, Cheetham T (2010) The use of psychotropic medication for the management of problem behaviours in adults with intellectual disabilities living in Canada. *Advances in Mental Health and Intellectual Disabilities* 4(3):12–26.

Deb S, Clarke D, Unwin G (2006) Using medication to manage behavioural problems in adults with learning disabilities. Birmingham: University of Birmingham. Available at: www.LD-Medication.bham.ac.uk (accessed 6 January 2015).

Frighi V, Stephenson MT, Morovat A, et al. (2011) Safety of antipsychotics in people with intellectual disability. *British Journal of Psychiatry* 1–7. Available at: http://bjp.rcpsych.org/content/early/2011/07/30/bjp.bp.110.085670.full.pdf (accessed 6 January 2015).

Griffiths H, Halder N, Chaudhry N (2012) Antipsychotic prescribing in people with intellectual disabilities: a clinical audit. *Advances in Mental Health and Intellectual Disabilities* 6(4):215–222.

Kalachnik JE, Leventhal BL, James DH, et al. (1998) Guidelines for the use of psychotropic medication. In: Reiss S, Aman MG, eds. *Psychotropic medication and developmental disabilities: the international consensus handbook.* Columbus: Ohio State University, Nisonger Centre, pp. 45–72.

Paton C, Flynn A, Shingleton-Smith A, et al. (2011) Nature and quality of antipsychotic prescribing practice in UK psychiatry of learning disability services: findings of a national audit. *Journal of Intellectual Disability Research* 55:665–674.

Rush AJ, Frances A (2000) Treatment of psychiatric and behavioural problems in mental retardation – expert consensus guideline series. *American Journal on Mental Retardation* 105(3):159–227.

Unwin GL, Deb S (2011) Efficacy of atypical antipsychotic medication in the management of behaviour problems in children with intellectual disabilities and borderline intelligence: a systematic review. *Research in Developmental Disabilities* 32(6):2121–2133.

Further reading

Deb S, Kwok H, Bertelli M, et al. (2009) International guide to prescribing psychotropic medication for the management of problem behaviours in adults with intellectual disabilities. *World Psychiatry* 8:181–186.

CHAPTER 3

Physical and Health Monitoring

David Branford[1] & Sabyasachi Bhaumik[2,3]

[1]*English Pharmacy Board, Royal Pharmaceutical Society, London, UK*
[2]*Leicestershire Partnership NHS Trust, Leicester, UK*
[3]*Department of Health Sciences, University of Leicester, Leicester, UK*

In England approximately 1.2 million people have learning disabilities (300,000 children, 900,000 adults).
They have significantly higher rates of mortality and morbidity than their non-learning disabled peers.
A significant proportion of this excess mortality and morbidity is avoidable, in the sense that effective health promotion, early diagnosis and good treatment could ameliorate it. This constitutes a health inequality.

Glover et al. (2012)

General physical monitoring

In 2008, Sir Jonathan Michael published a report in England called 'Healthcare for All', an independent inquiry into access to healthcare for people with intellectual disabilities. His primary finding was that people with intellectual disabilities find it much harder than other people to access assessment and treatment for general health problems that have nothing directly to do with their disability. His primary recommendation was that health organisations must secure general health services that make reasonable adjustments for people with intellectual disabilities through a direct enhanced service. In particular, enhanced primary care services that include regular health checks provided by GP practices and improve data, communication and cross-boundary partnership working must be commissioned.

The underlying rationale for the use of health checks has been summarised in the report of Glover et al. and a number of other reports:
- People with ID may be unaware of the medical implications of their symptoms, have difficulty communicating their symptoms or may be less likely to report them.
- Carers may not always attribute the symptoms to physical or mental illness.

The Frith Prescribing Guidelines for People with Intellectual Disability, Third Edition.
Edited by Sabyasachi Bhaumik, David Branford, Mary Barrett and Satheesh Kumar Gangadharan.
© 2015 John Wiley & Sons, Ltd. Published 2015 by John Wiley & Sons, Ltd.

- Primary care services are generally designed to be responsive to events or problems raised by people.
- Health checks provide a way to detect, treat and prevent new health conditions in the ID population.
- Health checks can help provide baseline information against which changes in health status can be monitored; this is particularly important if embarking on a treatment with medication.

In March 2013, the Royal College of Psychiatrists launched a programme called 'parity of esteem' from the report *Whole-Person Care: From Rhetoric to Reality. Achieving Parity between Mental and Physical Health* (Occasional Paper OP8). This paper emphasises the interconnection between physical well-being and mental health and vice versa.

The report stated that

> A 'parity approach' should enable NHS and local authority health and social care services to provide a holistic, 'whole person' response to each individual, whatever their needs, and should ensure that all publicly funded services, including those provided by private organisations, give people's mental health equal status to their physical health needs. Central to this approach is the fact that there is a strong relationship between mental health and physical health, and that this influence works in both directions. Poor mental health is associated with a greater risk of physical health problems, and poor physical health is associated with a greater risk of mental health problems. Mental health affects physical health and vice versa.

In England, guidance has been produced to help GPs, practice nurses and primary care teams organise and perform quality annual health checks on adults with an ID.

In addition, many of the medications prescribed for people with ID come with specific guidance on physical monitoring. This chapter largely focuses on such monitoring. Despite the emphasis on health checks, there is consistent concern that such monitoring is not being undertaken.

Key points specific to intellectual disability

Part 1: Methylphenidate
Introduction

Because of the chronic nature of ADHD, long-term treatment has been recommended in all ADHD treatment guidelines. Methylphenidate is the most commonly prescribed stimulant used to treat ADHD, with extended-release formulations available in many countries.

Treatment guidelines recommend routine monitoring for children treated with stimulant medications. Along with the regular assessments of treatment efficacy and the emergence of adverse effects, it has also been recommended that physicians routinely monitor height, weight, blood pressure (BP) and heart rate in people with ID treated with stimulants. In addition, routine haematologic monitoring, including periodic complete blood cell count, differential blood cell count and platelet counts, is advised during prolonged therapy with both immediate-release and extended-release methylphenidate formulations.

People with ID should be monitored for the risk of diversion, misuse and abuse of methylphenidate.

Part 2: Antipsychotic medication
Introduction
With greater clinical use of the atypical antipsychotics, there has been an awareness of their differing side effect profiles compared to the typical antipsychotics. Of particular concern is the increased risk of developing metabolic syndrome. This has highlighted the need to monitor the physical parameters in people with ID treated with antipsychotics.

Prevalence
Up to 25% of people with intellectual disability receive antipsychotics, and with the gradual change of prescribing, a large proportion will receive atypical antipsychotics. Much of the research relating to the prescribing of atypical antipsychotics and the metabolic syndrome has involved people with schizophrenia. A diagnosis of schizophrenia is an independent risk factor for diabetes and other aspects of the metabolic syndrome.

Atypical antipsychotics are also associated with weight gain in their own right. Whether having an intellectual disability also increases the risk of the metabolic syndrome is unclear. However:
- Various syndromes associated with ID are also associated with weight gain and altered cardiac profiles.
- Many people with ID receive other medications that are associated with weight gain.
- All antipsychotics have been associated with case reports of sudden onset of ketoacidosis and impaired glucose tolerance.

An audit was undertaken prospectively to examine the compliance of a group of psychiatrists against guidelines they had developed for monitoring the onset of metabolic syndrome. The audit used the set of standards on monitoring of the American Diabetes Association (2004).

Seventy-seven per cent of the psychiatrists felt that they did some baseline recording, but findings did not corroborate this – only 53.8% of the notes recorded the assessment of risk factors in personal history, 37.5% risk factors in family history, 31.7% baseline weight, and 26.4% baseline blood sugar/lipid levels.

Eighty-five per cent of the psychiatrists thought that they carried out some of the recommended monitoring, but the audit found the records of weight monitoring in 69.7% of the notes and blood sugar and lipids monitoring in 44.2%.

Teeluckdharry et al. (2013)

Cardiovascular risk history

It is important to take a detailed cardiovascular risk history before the decision to prescribe antipsychotics is made or as soon as clinically feasible after initiation. This is relevant given the current climate of uncertainty surrounding a possible link between certain antipsychotics and the observed incidence of stroke in certain individual with ID subsets. In the outpatient with ID setting, it may not be clinically appropriate in terms of engagement with the person with ID, or practicable, to request all cardiovascular monitoring parameters as a baseline.

It is suggested that baseline measurements of electrocardiogram (ECG), full fasting lipids and waist circumference are only necessary where there is evidence of increased cardiovascular risk from either personal or family history, body weight, or blood glucose result. Clinicians may wish to seek GP-held details of cardiovascular risk history. For people with ID living in institutional type settings, where there is easier access to monitoring facilities and increased potential for coexisting risk factors (such as more rapid dose escalation or agitation and hyperarousability in acute situations), it is recommended that all cardiovascular monitoring parameters be measured at or as close to baseline as is feasible.

Monitoring glucose control

Measuring random blood glucose is the most practical approach. Borderline results should be followed up by measuring a fasting blood glucose and proceeding to a glucose tolerance test if the fasting result so indicates. Glycosylated haemoglobin (HBA1c) provides a useful indication of glycaemic control over the preceding 4 months and can be used to track trends where uncertainty exists.

Hyperprolactinaemia

Raised serum prolactin (hyperprolactinaemia) is a well recognised side effect of antipsychotics. It can also be caused by other medications and by physiological disorders. The effect of raised prolactin varies from individual to individual and some people remain symptom-free. Concerns have been raised about potential long-term side effects, and there is a growing literature on this subject; however, currently, the research is inconclusive (Table 3.1).

There is a likely connection between high prolactin levels and osteoporosis, and bone health must be considered. Lifestyle advice on good calcium intake, exercise, stopping smoking and drinking alcohol is appropriate for all people with ID (Table 3.2).

Breast cancer

Concerns have been raised for many years about the possible link between circulating prolactin and breast cancer. The link remains uncertain. A recent retrospective cohort study found an increased risk of breast cancer in people with ID exposed to dopamine antagonists. Due to the small hazards and the possibility of residual confounding, it concluded that treatment strategies should not be changed. Further studies are required (Table 3.3).

Table 3.1 Causes of hyperprolactinaemia (not an exhaustive list).

Psychiatric medications	Non-psychiatric medications	Physiological disorders
Tricyclic antidepressants	Metoclopramide	Disorders of the hypothalamus, including tumours
MAOIs	Domperidone	Disorders of the pituitary, including tumours
Antipsychotics	Verapamil	Polycystic ovarian syndrome
More likely:	Methyldopa	Hypothyroidism
First-generation antipsychotics	Oestrogen	Renal failure
Risperidone	Opiates	Cirrhosis
Amisulpride		
Less likely:		
Aripiprazole		
Clozapine		
Olanzapine		
Quetiapine		

Table 3.2 Modifiable and non-modifiable risk factors associated with osteoporosis.

Modifiable risks	Non-modifiable risks
Smoking	Gender
Exercise	Age
Diet	Ethnicity
Alcohol	Family history of fractures
Hypogonadism	Personal history of fractures
Medication, for example, glucocorticoid therapy, anticonvulsants	

Table 3.3 Testing schedule for antipsychotics.

Test	Test interval
Body weight and body mass index (BMI)	Baseline, 3/12, 6/12 and then every 6/12
Blood pressure and pulse	Baseline, 3/12, 6/12 and then every 6/12
Urea and electrolytes (U&E)	Baseline, 3/12, 6/12 and then every 6/12
Liver function tests (LFTs)	Baseline, 3/12, 6/12 and then every 6/12
Full blood count (FBC)	Clozapine: as per manufacturers' guidelines
	Others: baseline, 3/12, 6/12 and then every 6/12
Blood glucose	Baseline, 3/12, 6/12 and then every 6/12
Thyroid function test (TFT)	Baseline and then annually
Prolactin	Baseline, repeat only if clinically indicated

Part 3: High doses of antipsychotics

Definition

A single antipsychotic prescribed at a daily dose above the British National Formulary (BNF)-recommended maximum dose or more than one antipsychotic – assessed by expressing the current dose of each antipsychotic as a percentage of the maximum BNF-recommended dose (or in the case of older adults, as a percentage of the recommended upper limit). Adding these together, more than 100% constitutes 'high dose'.

For example, zuclopenthixol depot 300 mg weekly and olanzapine 15 mg daily. In adult, $50 + 75\% = 125\%$. In older adult, $100 + 75\% = 175\%$.

NB: 'As-required' medication should be included.

The Royal College of Psychiatrists Consensus statement (May 2006) states:

> The essential message is that the use of high dose cannot be justified as a general clinical strategy, but equally the recognition that in a small proportion of cases such a practice could be justified, providing certain important procedures relating to safety and effectiveness are observed.

Potential high-dose antipsychotics

Many people with ID in addition to receiving regular antipsychotics also have antipsychotics (and other medications) prescribed to be available on an as-required or prn basis. This has led to very different accounts of the levels of antipsychotic high-dose treatment.

High-dose medication can be divided into two groups:

1 High dose of regular antipsychotic(s)

2 Potential high dose of regular and as-required (prn) antipsychotic(s) combined

It has been suggested that even in cases where there is only the occasional potential for high-dose antipsychotic (HDAT), the monitoring should be the same.

Prevalence of the use of HDAT in intellectual disability

There is a paucity of studies looking into the prevalence of use of HDAT in people with ID. Most of the studies have focused on the use of antipsychotics in the ID population in general, rather than specifically investigating the extent of antipsychotic polypharmacy or HDAT use. There have been a number of audits on this topic in different settings. The results vary:

• An audit on use of HDAT in an inpatient facility that included an admission and assessment unit, a medium secure forensic unit and a specialist unit for people with moderate to severe ID and challenging behaviours reported that 61% of the in-people with ID received two or more antipsychotics.

• A currently unpublished ID audit showed only 18 out of 1200 active inpatients and outpatients with ID in Leicestershire, England, satisfied the criteria of being on HDAT. Fifty per cent of this individual with ID population had the necessary investigations including an ECG. The authors concluded that the overall prevalence of use of single medication in high dose has reduced considerably.

- A similar unpublished audit in Lincolnshire, England, showed a prevalence rate of 7%. A community-based study in Nottinghamshire showed 3% on antipsychotics exceeded BNF limits and none of them had appropriate monitoring.

Factors influencing the use of HDAT

It has been suggested that there are three main factors that influence the prescribing of HDAT and antipsychotic polypharmacy: the person's clinical condition, psychiatrists' scepticism towards use of guidelines and algorithms and, finally, nurses' requests for more medication use.

Risks of HDAT/antipsychotic polypharmacy

People with ID may be more prone to adverse drug reactions (ADRs) than the general population due to a combination of factors such as the presence of brain damage, epilepsy, sensory deficits and physical health problems. However, as stated in the previous chapter, this remains controversial.

In adults with severe/profound ID who are more likely to suffer from concomitant physical health problems, including cardiac defects, use of HDAT or antipsychotic polypharmacy is not recommended. In rare circumstances when the use of HDAT or antipsychotic polypharmacy is thought to be the only option in the management of the underlying mental health problems in people with ID, the following suggestions should be followed to make a safer use of such an option:

- If HDAT or antipsychotic polypharmacy is to be used, this should be based on individual risk–benefit analysis and only considered after non-pharmacological and evidence-based pharmacological approaches have failed.
- The decision to prescribe must be made at a multidisciplinary level involving people with ID and carers. Issues in relation to capacity to consent should be addressed. If a decision to prescribe is made, clear plans should be in place for a specified period of trial with regular review arrangements. Clear documentation is a vital part of this process.
- Before starting an individual with ID on such a regime, any potential contraindications and interactions should be considered.
- Necessary physical examinations and baseline investigations, including an ECG, should be carried out prior to starting on the proposed regime and repeated as appropriate in short intervals, preferably every few weeks.
- Doses of medication should only be increased if absolutely necessary, and increases should be made slowly and not more often than once weekly.

Prescribing HDAT

Before prescribing high doses of antipsychotics, assess and consider:

- Compliance with treatment
- Sufficient time to respond
- Alternative antipsychotics, including clozapine
- Appropriateness of other adjunctive medications (e.g. mood stabilisers, antidepressants)

- Psychological approaches
- Risk factors (e.g. cardiac history, hepatic or renal impairment, tobacco or alcohol use, old age, obesity)
- Medication interactions

A second consultant opinion should be sought if there is no consensus of the benefit to the person with ID of continuing HDAT. If HDAT treatment is to continue after discharge or is initiated in the community, monitoring arrangements must be agreed and the GP should be informed.

Physical monitoring requirements may be carried out by the GP under the supervision of the consultant; however, responsibility for all aspects of treatment and associated management of people with ID receiving HDAT lies with the consultant psychiatrist overseeing the case.

If the individual with ID refuses or declines physical monitoring, this must be documented. The responsible prescriber must be informed and should, together with the individual with ID and their carer whenever possible, review and document risks and benefits of continuing HDAT treatment in coming to a decision about future treatment. The decision to refuse or decline physical monitoring and/or continue treatment without monitoring should be regularly reviewed with the individual with ID or carers as appropriate (minimum every 3 months).

The individual's progress should be reviewed at least 3-monthly, the dose reduced to within the licensed range if no significant progress is observed, and alternatives considered. After one year, if the individual with ID is stable, treatment is unchanging and there are no clinical indications for frequent monitoring, consider reducing physical monitoring (minimum annual review).

Unless otherwise stated, doses in the BNF are licensed doses – any higher dose is therefore unlicensed. The prescribing of licensed medication outside the recommendations of the marketing authorisation increases the prescriber's professional responsibility. The individual with ID or, if more appropriate, the carer should be informed that use is outside the licence. Always refer to the most up-to-date BNF in case of changes.

Although there is only one licensed maximum dose for each antipsychotic, it is strongly recommended to use the lower upper limit for older adults. Hence, when an antipsychotic dose falls between the licensed maximum dose and the recommended upper limit for older adults, these monitoring guidelines should be applied as they represent good clinical practice.

Physical monitoring advice

- Baseline ECG. If QTc is prolonged (>440 ms men, >470 ms women) or other abnormality develops, treatment should be reviewed and cardiology assessment considered.
- Repeat the ECG every few days during dose escalation.

- Monitor respiration, BP, pulse, temperature and fluid intake at least weekly initially.
- Check baseline urea and electrolytes (U&Es) and liver function test (LFTs).
- Repeat U&Es, BP, respiration, pulse, temperature and fluid intake 3-monthly.

Part 4: Mood stabilisers

In addition to the atypical antipsychotics, lithium and the antiepileptics sodium valproate, carbamazepine and lamotrigine are commonly prescribed as mood stabilisers. In ID, these medications have a multitude of indications. They include, in addition to the treatment and prophylaxis of bipolar illness, various unlicensed indications:

- Lithium for the management of aggression and self-injurious behaviour
- Carbamazepine for the management of aggression, self-mutilation, trigeminal neuralgia and epilepsy
- Sodium valproate for the management of migraine and epilepsy
- Lamotrigine for epilepsy and bipolar affective disorder

Regardless of the indication, monitoring is recommended. A testing regimen is advised in a number of key texts and in the standard product characteristics for each medication.

Key guidelines

SIGN Guideline No 52. (2001, June) Drug therapy with methylphenidate.

National Institute for Health and Clinical Excellence. (2009) Schizophrenia: core interventions in the treatment and management of schizophrenia in primary and secondary care (update). Clinical guideline 82. www.nice.org.uk/CG82 (accessed 6 January 2015)

National Institute for Health and Clinical Excellence. (2008) Lipid modification: cardiovascular risk assessment and the modification of blood lipids for the primary and secondary prevention of cardiovascular disease. Clinical guideline 67. www.nice.org.uk/CG67 (accessed 6 January 2015).

National Institute for Health and Clinical Excellence. (2004) Type 1 diabetes: diagnosis and management of type I diabetes in children, young people and adults. Clinical guideline 15. www.nice.org.uk/CG15 (accessed 6 January 2015).

National Institute for Health and Clinical Excellence. (2008) Type 2 diabetes: the management of type 2 diabetes (update). Clinical guideline 66. www.nice.org.uk/CG66 (accessed 6 January 2015).

National Institute for Health and Clinical Excellence. (2006) Obesity: guidance on the prevention identification, assessment and management of overweight and obesity in adults and children. Clinical guideline 43. www.nice.org.uk/CG43 (accessed 6 January 2015).

www.iassid.org/pdf/healthguidelines-2002.pdf (accessed 6 January 2015).

http://www.scotland.gov.uk/Publications/2013/06/1123/7 (accessed 6 January 2015).

The NHS Website for Primary Care Commissioning on the management of health for people with a learning disability. This site includes GP Information Systems e-templates for annual health checks and loading instructions. www.pcc.nhs.uk/management-of-health-for-people-with-learning-disabilities (accessed 6 January 2015).

References

American Diabetes Association, American Psychiatric Association, American Association of Clinical Endocrinologists, and North American Association for the Study of Obesity (2004) Consensus development conference on antipsychotic drugs and obesity and diabetes. *Diabetes Care* 27:596–601.

Glover, G, Emerson, E, Eccles, R (2012) *Using local data to monitor the health needs of people with learning disabilities.* Durham: Improving Health & Lives, Learning Disabilities Observatory.

Royal College of Psychiatrists (2006) *Consensus statement high-dose antipsychotic medication.* London: Royal College of Psychiatrists.

Teeluckdharry, S, Sharma, S, O'Rourke, E, et al. (2013) Monitoring metabolic side effects of atypical antipsychotics in people with an intellectual disability. *Journal of Intellectual Disabilities* 17(3):223–235.

Further reading

MENCAP (2007) Death by indifference. Report about institutional discrimination within the NHS, and people with a learning disability getting poor healthcare. www.mencap.org.uk/document.asp?id=284 (accessed 6 January 2015).

Robertson, J, Roberts, R, Emerson, E (2010) *Health checks for people with learning disabilities: a systematic review of evidence.* Durham: Improving Health & Lives, Learning Disabilities Observatory.

Royal College of Psychiatrists (2012) *Improving the health and wellbeing of people with learning disabilities: an evidence-based commissioning guide for Clinical Commissioning Groups (CCGs).* London: Royal College of Psychiatrists.

CHAPTER 4

Epilepsy

David Branford[1], Sabyasachi Bhaumik[2,3] & Reza Kiani[2]

[1]*English Pharmacy Board, Royal Pharmaceutical Society, London, UK*
[2]*Leicestershire Partnership NHS Trust, Leicester, UK*
[3]*Department of Health Sciences, University of Leicester, Leicester, UK*

> People think that epilepsy is divine simply because they don't have any idea what causes epilepsy. But I believe that someday we will understand what causes epilepsy, and at that moment, we will cease to believe that it's divine. And so it is with everything in the universe.
>
> *Hippocrates*

Definition

Epilepsy is a tendency to the occurrence of transient, recurrent, abnormal and unprovoked electrical discharges in the brain affecting one or more of the following brain functions: motor, sensory, autonomic, cognitive, speech, behaviour, emotions and psychological. Some specialists consider that a single seizure associated with electroencephalography (EEG) changes may have a high chance of recurrence and therefore be included in the definition of epilepsy.

The classification of seizures depends on whether the onset of the seizure begins locally or not, and on the nature of other symptoms and signs occurring during the seizure (Table 4.1). The distinction between simple and complex seizures based on whether consciousness is impaired or not during a seizure is contentious; the two are not easily distinguishable, particularly in those with limited speech.

Prevalence

Epilepsy is a common condition; in fact, it is the most common neurological condition worldwide. Studies in the general population show that the incidence rate is 50–70 per 100 000 people per year. The highest incidence rates are observed in

The Frith Prescribing Guidelines for People with Intellectual Disability, Third Edition.
Edited by Sabyasachi Bhaumik, David Branford, Mary Barrett and Satheesh Kumar Gangadharan.

Table 4.1 International classification of seizures.

Partial (focal) seizures (begin locally)	Simple partial seizures (consciousness not impaired)	With motor signs, for example, Jacksonian epilepsy (focal tonic spasm)
		With somatosensory or special sensory signs, for example, visual, auditory, olfactory, gustatory
		With autonomic signs or symptoms, for example, salivation, flushing, sweating, pallor
		With psychological symptoms, for example, perceptual or mood changes
	Complex partial seizures (with impaired consciousness)	• Beginning as a simple partial seizure (aura) and progressing to impaired consciousness
		• With focal motor signs
		• Gelastic seizures
		• Hemiclonic seizures
		• Focal negative myoclonus
		With impaired consciousness at outset: alone or with automatisms (psychomotor attacks), for example, lip-smacking, chewing, semi-purposeful behaviour
	Partial seizures evolving to secondarily generalised seizures	Simple partial seizures or complex partial seizures becoming tonic–clonic seizures
Generalised seizures (no local onset, bilaterally symmetrical)	Absence seizures (petit mal)	Typical absence seizures; 3 cycles/s spike and wave on EEG and 10–45 s lapse of consciousness
		Atypical absence seizures (often associated with an epileptic syndrome): 1–2.5/s spikes on EEG
	Myoclonic seizures	Sudden brief (<350 ms) stereotypical shock-like muscle contractions (any muscle group)
	Clonic seizures	Rhythmic or semi-rhythmic contractions of a group of muscles (any muscle group)
	Tonic seizures	Brief seizures (usually <60 s): sudden onset of increased tone in extensor muscles
	Tonic–clonic seizures (grand mal)	Generalised stiffening of flexor or extensor muscles (tonic phase) followed by generalised jerking of muscles (clonic phase)
	Atonic seizures (drop attacks)	Sudden loss in muscle tone → a drop attack
Unclassified	Any other seizures that do not fit into the above categories	

Source: International League Against Epilepsy (1981).
EEG, electroencephalography.

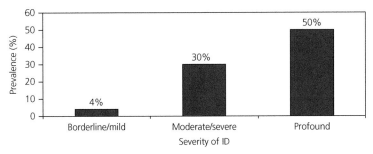

Figure 4.1 Prevalence of epilepsy in ID.

babies and young children and in older persons. The point prevalence rate is 0.5–1.0% a year. The lifetime risk for an individual developing epilepsy is 3–5%.

There is a greater prevalence of epilepsy in those with intellectual disability (ID) than in the general population. The exact prevalence of epilepsy in people with ID is difficult to estimate but varies between 14 and 24%. The prevalence depends on multiple factors including age, severity of ID and associated neurological conditions. The prevalence of epilepsy among people with mild to moderate ID is between 7 and 15%, among people with severe ID is about 67% and among people with profound ID varies between 50 and 82% (Figure 4.1). 10–20% of people with cerebral palsy have epilepsy compared to 50% of people with cerebral palsy and ID.

If an individual with severe ID has seizures at the age of 22, there is a 40% probability of seizures having been present for over 10 years. This indicates how chronic a condition epilepsy can be in people with ID.

The relationship between ID and epilepsy may be explained in a variety of ways:

Relationship between ID and epilepsy
- A brain abnormality leads to both ID and epilepsy, for example, perinatal trauma, encephalopathy, head injury, non-accidental injury, genetic syndrome (e.g. tuberous sclerosis), and neuro-migrational defects.
- Prolonged seizures during childhood may rarely cause reduced IQ, for example, febrile status epilepticus and hypsarrhythmia.
- Treatment of epilepsy may reduce IQ, for example, surgery and cognitive side effects of antiepileptics.
- Epilepsy and ID are present in one individual independently.

NB: Non-convulsive generalised status (e.g. absence status) may be mistaken for a low IQ, delirium or psychiatric/behavioural problems and can continue to be unrecognised for long periods of time.

Epidemiology of epilepsy in ID

Most studies have involved children with epilepsy and ID rather than adults. Key studies of the epidemiology of epilepsy in children with ID have found:
- Greater incidence of new cases appeared between ages 1 and 4 years.
- In children with an IQ lower than 50, one third had a history of seizures and 19% had at least one seizure during the previous year.

- By the age of 22, 15% of children with ID had epilepsy and an additional 7% had at least one seizure.
- Children with a history of postnatal injury suffered a much higher risk of epilepsy.

Despite this high prevalence of epilepsy, there are remarkably few studies of adults with ID. Key studies of the epidemiology of epilepsy in ID have found that there was no significant difference in the prevalence of epilepsy in South Asians and people with lightly pigmented skin. Studies in the general population have reported a higher prevalence of epilepsy in people with darkly pigmented skin.

Studies in the general population have reported a higher prevalence of epilepsy in lower socioeconomic groups. As most adults with ID have restricted opportunities for paid employment or car ownership and derive their income from state benefits, it is difficult to use indicators of socioeconomic groups in a meaningful way for internal comparisons.

Studies that have looked at the nature and course of the epilepsy in ID have found:

- The presence of both epilepsy and ID is an indicator of both early mortality and psychiatric disorder.
- The prevalence of epilepsy in ID remains constant for much of the period 20–60 years.

The nature of the epilepsy in adults with ID

Aetiology

The causes of epilepsy may be genetic, congenital or acquired (Table 4.2). However, in many patients, the cause is unknown (idiopathic). This is especially the case in people with mild ID where no aetiology for ID can be determined. A genetic abnormality may result in epilepsy alone or in epilepsy with other neurological manifestations as is found, for example, in Down syndrome and tuberous sclerosis. Many of the inborn errors of metabolism are associated with epilepsy. Most of these are very rare; and some are treatable, for example, phenylketonuria and pyridoxine deficiency. Susceptibility to recurrent infections and a lowering of the seizure threshold by certain medications may increase an individual's risk of developing epilepsy.

In about 20% of cases of ID, there is a genetic cause; in 30% of cases, the cause is prenatal; in 9–21% of cases, the cause is perinatal; and in 9–30% of cases, the cause is postnatal.

Certain causes of epilepsy are particularly likely to be related to development of epilepsy in childhood. Other causes are more likely to be associated with the development of epilepsy in adolescence. Causes such as the development of dementia in people with Down syndrome may be associated with

Table 4.2 Causes of epilepsy in people with ID.

Classification	Examples
Genetic	
Chromosomal abnormalities	Down syndrome
Dysplastic conditions	Tuberous sclerosis
	Sturge–Weber syndrome
	Megalencephaly
	Aicardi syndrome
Metabolic abnormalities	Phenylketonuria
	Maple syrup urine disease
	Pyridoxine deficiency
	Tay–Sachs disease
	Lipoidosis GM1 and GM3
	Metachromatic leucodystrophy
Congenital	
Dysplastic and neoplastic conditions	Cortical dysplasia or dysgenesis
	Cerebral tumours
Vascular malformations	Atrioventricular malformation
	Cavernous angioma
Perinatal injury	Antenatal brain injury
	Perinatal brain injury
Acquired	
Trauma and injury	Head injury – dural tear, depressed fracture, intracranial bleed, anoxia, neurosurgery
Prenatal infections	Cytomegalovirus
	Syphilis
	Toxoplasmosis
Postnatal infections	Purulent meningitis
	Acute encephalitis
	Subacute sclerosing panencephalitis
	Post-immunisation encephalopathy
	Post-traumatic infections
Metabolic disorders	Hepatic and renal disorders
	Hypoglycaemia and hyperglycaemia
	Hypocalcaemia and hypercalcaemia
	Anoxia
Toxic disorders	Alcohol or substance misuse
	Toxic effects of pharmacotherapy
	Lead
Vascular disease	Atherosclerosis
	Cardiovascular accident
Hippocampal sclerosis	Mesial temporal lobe epilepsy
Neurological degenerative disease	Dementia
Tumours and other space-occupying lesions	Cerebral tumours
	Cerebral abscesses

Table 4.3 Pathogenesis of the developmental causes of epilepsy.

Developmental process	Peak period	Results of abnormalities	Examples
Neuronal proliferation	2–4 months after conception	Microcephaly Macrocephaly	• Tuberous sclerosis
Neuronal migration	First 6 months of gestation	Generalised focal abnormalities: Pachygyria (gyri few and broad) Polymicrogyria (excessive small gyri)	• Heterotopia • Agenesis of the corpus callosum
Neuronal organisation	From 6th month of gestation to several years after birth	Abnormal neuronal organisation Abnormal neuronal layering Abnormal ramification of nerves Abnormal synaptic proliferation	• Rubella • Phenylketonuria • Down syndrome • West syndrome
Myelination	From 3rd month of gestation to maturity	Abnormal myelination	• Inborn errors of metabolism • Infections • Toxins • Alcohol • Hypoxia • Hypoglycaemia

even later development of epilepsy in adulthood. The most common cause of epilepsy in people with ID is developmental (Table 4.3). The brain passes through four main stages after the dorsal and ventral involutions of the embryonic neural plate, and at each stage, there is the potential for abnormalities to develop.

It should be emphasised that an episode of seizure in any person with or without a diagnosis of epilepsy should be fully investigated to rule out the treatable causes of seizures such as hypoglycaemia, hypocalcaemia and infection. In clinical practice, this is commonly seen in people with ID and epilepsy when a breakthrough seizure occurs suddenly in an otherwise well-controlled epileptic patient as a result of a urinary tract infection, menstruation, specific reflex triggers, flickering/flashing lights, non- or partial compliance or other identifiable medical triggers (medication and alcohol, insomnia and dehydration). In these circumstances, treatment of the underlying illness is the mainstay of treatment rather than increasing the dose of antiepileptic medication.

Frequency

The frequency of different seizure types in people with ID is detailed in Table 4.4. Thirty to forty per cent of adults with ID and epilepsy experience more than one seizure type, and 30–40% have more than one seizure per month.

Table 4.4 The frequency of seizure types in people with ID.

Seizure type	Prevalence (%)*
Tonic–clonic	60–83
Absences	15–37
Myoclonic/tonic/atonic (drop attack)	13–21
Partial seizure	25–28

*Some patients have more than one type of seizure.

Clinical presentation

Epilepsy is often difficult to diagnose in individuals with ID. They often have disordered cerebral anatomy or other cerebral pathology, which may alter the presentation of epilepsy. People with ID often lack the ability to give a subjective account of their seizures. For these reasons, good quality cerebral imaging such as magnetic resonance imaging (MRI) may be useful in helping to localise abnormalities. EEG and MRI can be offered to people with ID by well-trained staff that have the expertise to prepare and desensitise the clients for the procedures. Occasionally, sedation may be needed to carry out the procedure if clients are unable to cope in spite of all the support and preparation from the team. In this case, the risks and benefits of carrying out the procedure should be considered, including the likelihood of it changing the patient's management.

Many people with ID and epilepsy experience more than one type of seizure and some develop different types of epilepsy as they grow older. Although tonic–clonic seizures are the most common type of seizure in the ID population, absence seizures and myoclonic jerks occur more frequently than in the general population with epilepsy. Some other types of epilepsy are more common in people with ID. These include atonic, tonic and myoclonic epilepsies; the first two types make people with ID more prone to epilepsy-related injuries. People with ID due to their underlying brain damage suffer more from treatment-resistant epilepsy, and the presence of ID is a risk for sudden unexpected death in epilepsy (SUDEP). A recent study showed high SUDEP mortality rate in this population in comparison to the general population and no evidence that this subject had been discussed with the patients and their carers.

Differential diagnoses

Many other phenomena that occur in this population may be mistaken for epilepsy, and therefore, care should be taken not to diagnose epilepsy without enough convincing clinical information (e.g. sudden-onset episode, self-remitting in few minutes, aura, cliché-like attacks along with other seizure markers like sustaining injuries, incontinence, being unable to communicate during the attacks, post-ictal confusion).

Some examples of these differential diagnoses are:
- Abnormal posture (opisthotonus) and dystonias
- Parkinsonian side effects of psychotropic medications
- Non-epileptic attack (NEA) disorders
- Syncope
- Cardiac arrhythmias
- Cardiovascular disorder that present with orthostatic hypotension and fall
- Transient ischaemic attacks
- Migraine
- Cataplexy
- Episodic dyscontrol attacks
- Tics
- Hysterical fugue
- Transient global amnesia
- Peripheral nerve entrapment
- Transient vestibular symptoms
- Stereotypical autistic behaviours
- Eye movements disorders, eye deviation and nystagmus
- Respiratory phenomena such as obstructive sleep apnoea, hyperventilation and periodic breathing
- Metabolic problems (hypoglycaemia, hypocalcaemia, etc.)
- Anxiety disorders (e.g. panic attacks)
- Hyperekplexia (abnormal startle response)
- Non-epileptic myoclonic phenomena
- Gastro-oesophageal reflux (Sandifer's syndrome)
- Abnormal EEG in the context of an underlying brain damage or autism
- Parasomnias

NEA

NEA are described as paroxysmal events that can be mistaken for epilepsy. Their causes include physiological and psychological. Physiological causes are multiple, including metabolic imbalances, migraine, vertigo, TIAs, rhythmic movement disorders, acute dystonic reactions, cardiac arrhythmias and vasovagal syncope, among others. Psychogenic NEA have been previously described as psychogenic epilepsy or pseudoseizures. The true prevalence of NEA is unknown; however, they account for 20–30% of individuals referred for suspected epilepsy and 10–30% of those with active epilepsy.

NEA of psychogenic origin may present atypically and include usually prolonged and frequent attacks in spite of normal EEG findings, a fluctuating course, attacks with gradual onset, violent thrashing and flailing movements, side-to-side head movements, pelvic thrusting and opisthotonus. Attacks usually occur in public places/in front of witnesses; there may be apparent preservation of awareness; eyes may be shut with resistance to open them. Tongue biting and significant injuries are usually uncommon though may happen; however, friction (carpet) burns may be seen. There is usually an association with secondary gain, which can be identified with careful history taking. A past history of abuse may be present.

NEA of psychogenic origin is a diagnosis of exclusion; however, video telemetry at the time of attacks showing a normal EEG can help confirm the diagnosis, although it should be remembered that certain types of true epileptic seizure, such as frontal lobe seizures, do not always show up on EEG. In addition, it should be remembered that NEA of psychogenic origin can coexist with true epilepsy.

Whatever the cause of NEA, the main therapeutic issue is to avoid further harm through incorrect diagnosis and antiepileptic drug (AED) treatment. Psychological management is the mainstay of treatment for NEA of psychogenic origin, and drug treatment is not recommended.

Epilepsy and autism

A considerable number of people with ID plus autism develop epilepsy during their lifetime, but the prevalence rate varies across studies due to the heterogeneity of this population and the different methodologies and sample population studied. Autism seems to be the final presentation of a variety of abnormalities of brain development that are also seen in people with epilepsy. Autism and epilepsy can share a common genetic or neurodevelopmental cause; equally, it has been shown that epilepsy itself may induce the development of autism.

The term 'syndromal autism' has been used to describe those people with autism and associated neurodevelopmental syndromes. Syndromal autism has been found to be significantly associated with a higher female-to-male ratio, low IQ, more seizures and abnormal EEGs and more brain abnormalities on MRI. A meta-analysis on autism and epilepsy found a strong discrepancy in relative risk (RR) according to IQ, with more autistic patients with ID having epilepsy. The results of this meta-analysis indicated that risk for epilepsy in autism was higher in people with severe ID and female patients.

Epilepsy and Down syndrome

Although the prevalence of seizures in people with Down syndrome varies across different studies, approximately 10% of adults with Down syndrome develop epilepsy, increasing to 25–40% of those over the age of 40, being higher in those with Alzheimer's disease. Seizure types commonly seen in people with Down syndrome are tonic–clonic, myoclonic, startle and reflex epilepsy, focal and complex seizures and infantile spasms. EEG findings can vary extensively from no abnormalities to hypsarrhythmia.

There are three peaks in the incidence of epilepsy during the lifespan of an individual with Down syndrome:

1 In early childhood, there is a particular association between epilepsy and West syndrome. In those with Down syndrome, West syndrome is more benign, with more myoclonic seizures and more easily controlled than in those without Down syndrome.

2 During the third decade of life, a rise in epilepsy among people with Down syndrome appears to be the equivalent of the increased incidence of partial epilepsies seen in adolescent individuals without ID. This is thought to be related to myelination and proliferation of a sufficient bulk of nerves and synapses to connect abnormal areas of brain and thus allow paroxysmal spread.

3 Epilepsy in Down syndrome finally peaks with the development of Alzheimer's disease in those over the age of 40. In 60% of individuals, seizures start after the clinical onset of dementia. The seizures are usually tonic–clonic, although myo-clonic seizures may be particularly prominent.

In addition to these increased incidences of epilepsy in Down syndrome, certain forms of epilepsy are less common than might be expected. For example, despite the increased incidence of infections in infants with Down syndrome, febrile con-vulsions are rare. There is also a lower incidence of Lennox–Gastaut syndrome, an important cause of severe epilepsy in people with ID.

The mechanisms by which epilepsy is generated in Down syndrome are not entirely clear, although it has been suggested that the following characteristics of the brain are relevant:

• A small brain with abnormal neocortical cytoarchitecture
• Reduced number of granule cells – possibly inhibitor GABA cells
• Abnormal morphology of neurones and dendrites – which may enhance excitability
• Altered neuronal physiology and membrane reactivity
• Neurotransmitter abnormalities such as of glutamate

It should be remembered that there are a variety of causes of 'funny turns' in people with Down syndrome, including breath-holding, behaviour disturbance, cardiac dysrhythmias, sleep disorders and many undiagnosable episodes. Therefore, careful assessment with observation, electroencephalography (EEG) and MRI scanning is vital.

Epilepsy in Down syndrome responds well to antiepileptic medication, and therefore, the prognosis is good except in those with Alzheimer's dementia. The choice of antiepileptic depends on the type of seizure, but generally, broad-spectrum antiepileptic medications are effective. Diagnosis of epilepsy is clinical, and hence, the whole range of investigations may not be appropriate for people with dementia, especially complex procedures like EEG and computerised tomography/magnetic resonance imaging (CT/MRI) scans, which may cause more distress to the service users than any benefits. Other aspects of investiga-tions such as a full physical examination and blood tests should always be considered.

Other syndromes associated with ID and epilepsy

In addition to the classification of seizures, there is a separate system for epilepsies and epileptic syndromes. An epilepsy syndrome is a collection of characteristic clinical features that relate to a cluster of symptoms and signs. Syndromes are defined by seizure type(s), age of onset of seizures, aetiology, seizure-provoking factors, developmental status, EEG findings, genetics and neuroimaging.

Epilepsy syndromes are divided into:
- Localisation-related or focal epilepsies (those with partial-onset seizures)
- Generalised epilepsies (those with generalised seizures)

Based on the knowledge of aetiology, the syndromes are then further subdivided into:
- Idiopathic – presumed to be genetic in origin
- Symptomatic (secondary) – of known cause
- Cryptogenic – presumed to be symptomatic but with an unidentified underlying abnormality

---

The advantages of a syndrome diagnosis, as opposed to seizure diagnosis only, are that it provides much more information, including:
- Predicted prognosis, not only from the point of view of the epilepsy but also in relation to other features such as learning and behaviour
- Treatment selection: the choice of treatment may not only depend on seizure type but also the syndrome
- Defining the likelihood of underlying diagnosis
- Genetic counselling, where appropriate

Individuals with ID are more likely to have associated syndromal diagnosis; or in some cases, epilepsy and ID can be both part of a syndrome, such as Lennox–Gastaut and Rett syndrome.

Table 4.5 details some of the common epilepsy syndromes that occur in association with ID.

Approximately a quarter of patients with fragile X syndrome have accompanying epilepsy, and this association is more common in males than in females with this syndrome. In genetic syndromes that can cause severe to profound ID (e.g. Aicardi, Rett, Angelman), the prevalence of epilepsy can increase to 80–90%, which in the majority of the cases is treatment resistant. Neurocutaneous syndromes such as tuberous sclerosis and Sturge–Weber syndromes are also commonly associated with epilepsy.

Epilepsy, mental ill health and behaviour disorders

Behaviour problems and psychiatric illnesses are often seen in conjunction with epilepsy in people with ID and pose a management challenge for clinicians in their day-to-day practice. It is therefore important to find out whether there is any relationship between these and the epilepsy or its management.

Table 4.5 Epilepsy syndromes associated with ID.

Syndrome	Common characteristics	Age of onset	Degree of LD	Seizure type	Treatment choice	Prognosis
Aicardi syndrome	• Only occurs in girls • Structural brain abnormalities, with absence of the corpus callosum • Abnormalities of the retina • Physical abnormalities	Before 3 months of age	Severe	• Infantile spasms (West syndrome) Less likely: • Partial motor and complex partial seizures	Depending on the seizure type: • Vigabatrin • Corticosteroids may be helpful	Treatment resistant May die before early adulthood
Angelman syndrome	• Speech delay • Abnormality on chromosome 15	Between 18 months and 2 years of age	Moderate to mild	• Myoclonic jerks • Atonic • Tonic • Generalised tonic–clonic • Prolonged absences	• Sodium valproate • Lamotrigine • Carbamazepine • Levetiracetam	Epilepsy improves with time, usually after 10 years of age and may disappear completely by 10–12 years
Benign myoclonic epilepsy in infancy	• More common in boys than girls • Familial link	From 4 months to 3 years of age	Some have normal intellectual development, but some risk of delayed learning	• Brief, with head nodding, arm elevation, leg flexion and loss of balance	• Sodium valproate	
Early myoclonic encephalopathy	• Possible underlying biochemical disorder • Multiple aetiology; metabolic, migration disorder, non-ketotic hyperglycinaemia • Frequent seizures • After several months of seizures usually changes to West syndrome • Neurological abnormalities floppy • Many familial cases	New born or very early infancy	Severe	• Myoclonic jerks • Massive myoclonic movements • Partial motor seizures • Tonic spasms	• Phenobarbital • Corticosteroids **Do not use sodium valproate**	Treatment resistant May die within first year of life

Syndrome	Features	Age	Severity	Seizure types	Treatment	Prognosis
Epilepsy with myoclonic absences	• More common in boys • Familiar link		Varying degrees	• Severe rhythmical jerking to upper limbs • Tonic–clonic seizures • Atonic seizures • Typical absence seizures	• Sodium valproate • Ethosuximide • Lamotrigine • Clobazam	May be treatment resistant
Generalised epilepsy with febrile seizure plus	• Familial link • Start with febrile convulsions, and continue over the normal age range • Seizures associated with fever	6 months to 6 years of age	Varying degrees	• Febrile seizures • Febrile seizures plus (beyond normal age range) • Afebrile generalised tonic–clonic seizures • Absence seizures • Myoclonic seizures • Atonic seizures • Partial seizures	Depending on seizure type: • Febrile seizures: not required • Sodium valproate • Lamotrigine • Ethosuximide • Clobazam	May require a combination of medications Depends on seizure type, may stop at the age of 6, but can be lifelong
Lennox–Gastaut syndrome	• Frequent seizures • May have identified cause, for example, tuberous sclerosis • Proceeded by West syndrome in 20% • Behavioural disturbances • Epilepsy slows – psychic disorders worsen	2–8 years of age	Moderate to severe	• Atonic seizures • Absence seizures • Non-convulsive status epilepticus • Tonic seizures • Tonic–clonic seizures • Partial motor seizures • Complex partial seizures • Myoclonic seizures	• Sodium valproate • Lamotrigine • Topiramate • Clobazam • Phenytoin • Ketogenic diet • Corpus callosotomy • Vagus nerve stimulation	May be treatment resistant

(Continued)

Table 4.5 (*Continued*)

Syndrome	Common characteristics	Age of onset	Degree of LD	Seizure type	Treatment choice	Prognosis
Migrating partial epilepsy in infancy	• Start infrequently but progress up to 50 times a day, every day	First weeks of life, but by 6 months of age	Severe	• Partial seizures • Tonic–clonic seizures	• Ketogenic diet • Possibly bromide	Treatment resistant
Myoclonic–astatic epilepsy	• More common in boys • Familial link • Normal development and neurology	One to 5 years of age	Severe	• Atonic • Myoclonic • Absences • Tonic–clonic	• Sodium valproate • Lamotrigine • Clobazam • Ethosuximide	May be treatment resistant in 50%
Ohtahara syndrome	• Underlying structural brain abnormality • Genetic link • After several months may change to West syndrome • Neurologically very abnormal	Before 3 months of age, usually in first 10 days of life	Severe	• Tonic spasms • Partial motor seizures	• Surgery	Treatment resistant Often die within first 2 years of life
Rasmussen's syndrome (sometimes called Kojewnikow's syndrome)	• Chronic localised encephalitis (although no virus has been isolated) • Slow progressive neurological deficit	Anytime in childhood	Severe	• Focal seizures • Epilepsia partialis continua	• Surgery	Treatment resistant Short lifespan
Rett syndrome	• Boys are always affected more severely than girls • Genetic link in X chromosome • Normal development in first 6 to 18 months	After 2 years of age	Severe	• Tonic–clonic seizures • Absence seizures • Myoclonic seizures • Tonic seizures • Infantile spasms	• Sodium valproate • Carbamazepine • Lamotrigine • Clobazam	Difficult to treat May become less problematic in adolescence Shortened lifespan

Syndrome	Features	Onset	Severity	Seizure types	Treatment	Prognosis
Severe myoclonic epilepsy in infancy	• Only recently described • May start with seizures similar to febrile seizures • May be triggered by hot environments	First year of life	Severe	• Partial seizures • Myoclonic jerks • Very photosensitive • Febrile convulsions • Absences	• Phenobarbital • Sodium valproate • Topiramate • Clonazepam • Clobazam • Ketogenic diet **Lamotrigine: may make myoclonic seizures worse**	Treatment resistant
Sturge–Weber syndrome	• Presence of a birthmark, port wine stain • Very, very rare • Seizures develop in 2/3 of all children • Glaucoma • Hemiplegia	At birth or later in the first year of life	Severe	• Partial motor seizures • Atonic seizures • Myoclonic seizures • Infantile spasms • Frequent and prolonged seizures, resulting in status epilepticus. Todd's paralysis on recovery	• Surgical treatment: Hemispherectomy or hemispherotomy	Treatment resistant
West syndrome	• May be initially mistaken as colic • Clusters of seizures • Rapid breathing leading to fainting that may be misinterpreted as seizures • Arrhythmia • Brain malformations • Metabolic disorders • 90% have infantile spasms	Between 3 months and 1 year of age	Severe	• Sudden flexion, symmetrical	• Steroids • Vigabatrin • Nitrazepam • Sodium valproate	May be treatment resistant Most go on to develop other forms of seizures including Lennox–Gastaut syndrome

It is also important to emphasise that although majority of psychotropic medications are known to lower the seizure threshold, these do not cause significant concerns clinically, and concomitant mental health problems should be effectively treated. Risk of suicide is higher in people who have epilepsy; therefore, this needs to be assessed routinely in patients. On the other hand, some antiepileptics may have adverse effect on mental health, and some might particularly increase the chance of psychiatric illness or challenging behaviour (either as a result of their direct side effects or rarely through the process of forced normalisation). Therefore, interaction of these medications can cause a very confusing picture clinically, which can be compounded by the fact that often these patient groups are on other types of medication due to high prevalence of medical co-morbidities. The psychosocial impact of epilepsy (e.g. stigma, not being able to drive or pursue some leisure activities), genetic vulnerability and underlying aetiology of epilepsy are other causes of increased co-morbidity of mental health problems in this population. When treating psychiatric disorders in people who have epilepsy, the same biopsychosocial strategies that are used in the general population should be used, in order to achieve a better outcome.

Psychiatric illnesses in the context of epilepsy can be classified into different categories based on their presentation in relation to the time of the seizure: pre-ictally, ictally, post-ictally and inter-ictally. For a detailed review of these associations, readers are advised to refer to the neuropsychiatry of epilepsy by Trimble and Schmitz (2011).

Investigations

Diagnosis of epilepsy remains a clinical one. Various investigations such as MRI and EEG are used to support the diagnosis. The investigation of epilepsy in adults with ID will depend on the clinical picture presented and the practicality of carrying out the chosen tests in the individual concerned. The following list of investigations provides a format for considering what may be appropriate for a particular patient.

Hierarchy of investigations for epilepsy in adults with ID
- Clinical:
  - Seizure history
  - Seizure observation, including video recording
  - Physical examination, including blood pressure
  - Laboratory:
    - Blood testing for seizure causes and baseline prior to treatment
    - Consider urine analysis for detecting metabolic disorders

- Cardiological:
  - Electrocardiogram (ECG) for cardiac causation
  - Consider tilt test in suspected syncope
- Neurophysiological:
  - Inter-ictal EEG (with or without hyperventilation and photosensitivity)
  - Sleep and ambulatory EEG
  - EEG video telemetry (gold standard)
- Radiological:
  - Brain CT/MRI
- Specialist investigations (prior to neurosurgery):
  - Intracranial and cortical EEG
  - Deep brain EEG and stimulation
  - Diffusion tensor imaging (DTI) and MRS
  - Electroencephalography-correlated functional magnetic resonance imaging (EEGfMRI)
  - Single-photon emission computed tomography (SPECT) (subtraction of inter-ictal from ictal) and positron emission tomography (PET)
  - Magneto-encephalography (MEG)

EEG monitoring in people with ID

The process of carrying out an EEG in a person with ID, as indeed any of these investigations, may require considerable preparation, time and patience. The benefits and pitfalls of undertaking EEG monitoring, including the likelihood of the findings impacting on the person's management, need to be considered before undertaking the test. The following should be considered when interpreting the nature and significance of EEG findings in a person with ID:

- Abnormalities will be present in 72–91% of EEG recordings.
- Between 47 and 64% show excessive slow background activity.
- About 42% show epileptiform abnormalities.
- 18–22% show focal epileptiform activity.

Illustrative case study 4.1

A 30-year-old woman with mild ID and a diagnosis of tonic–clonic seizures who was seizure-free for a number of years on a combination of sodium valproate and carbamazepine presented with a 6-month history of episodic self-remitting bizarre behaviours. These lasted a few minutes and occurred two to three times per week. They were originally thought to be behavioural in nature. These were unresponsive to psychosocial strategies and environmental adaptations, therefore raising the suspicion of a newly diagnosed complex partial epilepsy. However, there was no response to an increased dose of carbamazepine. A brain MRI scan revealed a well-demarcated meningioma in the frontal lobe (her previous brain MRI about 10 years ago had been reported normal), which was successfully resected without complication. Following operation, seizure control improved considerably.

Table 4.6 Examples of epilepsy-related death.

- Drowning, burn injuries and falls/head trauma
- Sudden unexpected death in epilepsy
- Suicide
- Side effects or toxicity of AEDs
- Consequence of surgical treatment of epilepsy
- Foreign bodies aspiration/choking during a seizure

Epilepsy mortality

Mortality rate in people with epilepsy and ID is several times higher than the general population. A recent study revealed that all-cause-specific standardised mortality rates (SMRs) were 2.2 (95% confidence interval (CI), 2.0–2.4) and 2.8 (95% CI, 2.5–3.1) for men and women with ID, respectively. SMRs were 3.2 (95% CI, 2.7–3.8) and 5.6 (95% CI, 4.6–6.7) for men and women with epilepsy and ID, respectively.

Table 4.6 provides information on different epilepsy-related causes of death in people with ID.

SUDEP

SUDEP accounts for 7–17% of epilepsy-related deaths. In patients with ID and severe epilepsy, SUDEP is probably the most common cause for seizure-related deaths. Incidence data on SUDEP varies based on the cohort studied. A study of patients in the community prescribed antiepileptic medications showed an incidence of approximately 1:1000/year. The incidence of SUDEP in people with ID and epilepsy is estimated at 1:295/year. A recent study calculated the SMRs for SUDEP in patients with ID and found that these were 37.6 for men (95% CI, 21.9–60.2) and 52.0 for women (95% CI, 23.8–98.8). However, these figures might be an underestimate, as inaccurate death certificate classification has resulted in significant under-reporting of cases of SUDEP. The study also found that in the majority of ID cases, there was little detailed documentation on the circumstances surrounding death, no communication with patients/carers about risk of death in epilepsy and an absence of post-mortem reports or carers' referral for bereavement counselling.

Following a UK national audit undertaken by the National Institute for Health and Clinical Excellence (NICE) in 2002, it was estimated that 59% of child SUDEP deaths and 39% of adult SUDEP deaths were potentially or probably avoidable with adequate medication management. SUDEP has been shown to be associated with the following risk factors:
- Demographic:
  - Most cases of SUDEP have been observed in patients with epilepsy aged 20–40 years. The mean age is estimated to be 28.6 years. SUDEP is rare in children.

- Male-to-female ratio as high as 7:4 has been reported in most studies.
- African Americans have higher rates of SUDEP, but this may be due to the higher rate of epilepsy in this population.
- Other risk factors:
  - ID increases the risk of SUDEP.
  - Excessive alcohol consumption is a more frequent behaviour in patients with SUDEP than in the general population of patients with epilepsy.
- Epilepsy:
  - Symptomatic seizures are reported in 34–70% of SUDEP cases. Generalised tonic–clonic seizures, lower age of onset of seizures, duration of seizure disorder longer than 10 years and history of therapeutic surgery for epilepsy are other seizure-related risk factors. Most patients who die of SUDEP had poorly controlled seizures.
  - In a population of patients with refractory epilepsy who underwent therapeutic surgery, only patients who continued to have seizures were at risk for SUDEP. No patients who became seizure-free after surgery died.
- Medication:
  - Levels of AEDs at post-mortem have been shown to be sub-therapeutic in most cases of SUDEP. This might be due to poor compliance with AEDs, which is common in SUDEP.
  - Patients on multiple AEDs had a significantly higher rate of SUDEP than patients with epilepsy maintained on a single AED.
  - Recent change in AED therapy has also been implicated.

Advice to clinicians

Patient education plays a significant role in preventing sudden death. Sufficient information is now available to reassure most patients, identify high-risk patients and suggest means to reduce risk of SUDEP. The issue of SUDEP needs to be discussed specifically with patients and caregivers. Optimal seizure management with effective monotherapy and therapeutic levels of AEDs should be the aim of epilepsy management. Caregivers need to be trained in the acute management of tonic–clonic seizures, use of emergency medication to abort seizures and other practical approaches, including positioning the patient during and after the attack and delivering cardiopulmonary resuscitation.

Respiration needs to be monitored during the post-ictal period. Stimulating the person post-ictally is believed to reduce the chances of apnoea related to SUDEP. SUDEP is far more common in an outpatient setting than in a group home setting where the staff have received training in first aid treatment of tonic–clonic seizures. Compliance with medication and extra care and monitoring when switching AEDs is vital.

Epilepsy management

NICE guidance

National guidance on the management of epilepsy in adults with ID in the UK was updated by NICE in 2012 (CG137). Some of the keys points from this document are summarised in the following table (Table 4.7). The original text is a good source for those who wish to learn more about the holistic management of epilepsy.

The epilepsy care plan

One of the key messages from the NICE guideline is that epilepsy in the ID population should be managed with a biopsychosocial approach, through a multidisciplinary and multiagency process. An important tool for this approach is the production of a comprehensive epilepsy care plan, with a minimum annual review. An overview of the epilepsy care plan can be seen in Table 4.8, with further information on certain aspects discussed in more detail later in the chapter.

Recording of seizures: The seizure diary

To provide good management, it is vital to have a good recording system in place. A seizure diary should include clear descriptions of the following:
* The types of seizures that have occurred, described in simple language rather than in medical terms
* The frequency and duration of each seizure
* Records of any prolonged seizure necessitating administration of rescue medication (e.g. buccal midazolam) or emergency services intervention

There should also be clear records of the response to a new medication, including the impact on a patient's activities and behaviours and any medication side effects.

Table 4.7 Summary of NICE guidance of epilepsy in people with ID.

* Patient should have access to a specialist epilepsy clinic within 2 weeks if epilepsy is suspected
* Every therapeutic option should be explored in children, young people and adults with epilepsy in the presence or absence of ID
* Children, young people and adults with ID should not be discriminated against and must be offered the same services, investigations and therapies as for the general population
* Those with ID may require particular attention to tolerate investigations
* Facilities should be available for imaging under anaesthesia, if necessary
* Investigations directed at determining an underlying cause should be undertaken
* Adequate time for consultation should be offered to achieve effective management of epilepsy
* The patient and their family and/or carers should be enabled to take an active part in developing a personalised care plan for treating their epilepsy while taking into account any co-morbidities
* In making a care plan, particular attention should be paid to the possibility of adverse cognitive and behavioural effects of AED therapy
* The recommendations on choice of treatment and the importance of regular monitoring of effectiveness and tolerability are the same for those with ID as for the general population

Table 4.8 Areas of focus within an epilepsy care plan.

Biological
1. Diagnosis and aetiology of seizures
2. Seizure type, severity and frequency (review of seizure diary – see below)
3. Presence and management of prolonged seizures
4. Review of co-morbidities
5. Benefits, side effects and possible interactions of medications

Psychosocial
6. Full exploration of therapeutic options
7. Review of lifestyle issues (employment, ability for independent living, contraception, etc.)
8. Carer education and training

Risk assessment: Comprehensive risk assessment (see below)
Plan: Need for further investigations, medication changes or involvement of other agencies

As well as an awareness of the current clinical picture, it is vital for clinicians working in this field to obtain a thorough understanding of a patient's baseline seizure history. For example, a patient's epilepsy control may appear very poor while actually being at its best when the previous treatment-resistant history is known about. Therefore, always ask the carers if the seizure control currently is the same, better or worse than in the past. Having said that, it is also paramount to aspire to an ideal seizure control and never assume that someone with ID cannot be seizure-free.

Risk assessment

A good risk assessment is another vital part of the epilepsy review. Particular areas to focus on within the risk assessment include:
- Risks in the home – particularly the kitchen, bathroom (bathing) and stairs
- Risks within the community – particularly the risk of falls (which could potentially be ameliorated by a wheelchair or protective helmet, provided after physiotherapy input)
- Risks related to leisure activities – particularly swimming or cycling

It is important to check that patients with severe intractable epilepsy (especially tonic–clonic epilepsy) have an easily accessible protocol for the use of rescue medication during an emergency. The Joint Epilepsy Council has developed guidelines for use of rectal diazepam and buccal midazolam as rescue medications (www.jointepilepsycouncil.org.uk).

Principles of pharmacotherapy

The main goals of medication treatment in epilepsy are:
1 To achieve control of or, ideally, freedom from seizures. In the management of epilepsy in someone with accompanying damage or abnormal structure of the brain, the latter is not often possible.

2 To maintain a quality of life that allows the individual to participate meaning-
fully in day-to-day activities. This is mainly related to the tolerability and the
side effects of AEDs in practice.

These two goals need to be balanced as full control of seizures is not always
possible.

Starting treatment

AED treatment should only be started after full consideration of the risks and
benefits. The decision should be made after discussion with the person and their
family/carers. Treatment is generally recommended after a second epileptic seizure;
however, it may be considered after the first unprovoked seizure if:

- The person has a neurological deficit
- Brain imaging shows a structural abnormality
- The EEG shows unequivocal epileptic activity
- Having a second seizure is not acceptable for the patient or the family/carer
  (NICE, 2012)

In people with ID, it is better to start AED treatment at a lower dose than the BNF
recommendation and to titrate the dose up more slowly. If a second AED is needed,
it should be introduced slowly and attempts made to try and very gradually withdraw the first medication once the optimum dose of the second medication is
reached. Only one medication should be added or withdrawn at any one time, and
the aim should be to use monotherapy whenever possible.

In some people with ID or autism, tablets may not be accepted easily; therefore, other forms of medication such as syrup or powder are more appropriate,
although this might adversely affect the treatment cost.

Covert administration of medication

In some patients, there is no option except to administer medication covertly
mixed with food or drink. It is advisable to discuss this with the local pharmacist to ensure that efficacy is maintained by mixing it with a suitable food or
drink item (e.g. not mixing with a hot drink or just sprinkling the powder on
top of yogurt).

If covert medication is used, it is paramount that the correct legal frame-
works (e.g. Mental Capacity Act) and national guidelines are followed, to
demonstrate that the team has acted in the best interest of the patient in order
to avoid the serious morbidity and mortality potentially caused by
noncompliance.

The multidisciplinary team (MDT) should discuss in detail the risks and
benefits of covert administration of medication with full involvement of the
carers, the families and the patient's advocate (or independent mental capacity
advocate) or legal representative of the patient if already involved. Detailed
record-keeping should be put in place to safeguard the patient as well as the
professionals concerned.

Antiepileptic medications (AEDs)

Choice of antiepileptics

Choice of AED depends on the type of seizure (Tables 4.9 and 4.10). Although a number of new AEDs have been introduced, NICE still recommends carbamazepine and sodium valproate as first line. However, with both of these medications, certain client groups will be unsuitable. For example, sodium valproate should be

Table 4.9 Medication treatment for different types of epilepsy: Partial seizures.

Type of seizure	First-line medications	Adjunctive medications
Simple partial seizures	Carbamazepine	Gabapentin
Complex partial seizures	Sodium valproate	Tiagabine
Partial seizures evolving to secondarily generalised seizures	Lamotrigine	Levetiracetam
	Oxcarbazepine	Clobazam
	Levetiracetam	Zonisamide
		Topiramate
		Lacosamide
		Pregabalin
		Eslicarbazepine

Table 4.10 Medication treatment for different types of epilepsy: Generalised seizures.

Type of seizure	First-line medications	Adjunctive medications
Absence seizures (petit mal)	Sodium valproate	Lamotrigine
	Lamotrigine	Sodium valproate
	Ethosuximide	Ethosuximide
		Topiramate
		Clobazam
		Clonazepam
		Zonisamide
Myoclonic seizures	Sodium valproate	Sodium valproate
	Topiramate	Topiramate
	Levetiracetam	Clonazepam
		Levetiracetam
		Piracetam
		Clobazam
		Zonisamide
Tonic seizures and atonic seizures (drop attacks)	Sodium valproate	Topiramate
		Lamotrigine
		Rufinamide
Tonic–clonic seizures (grand mal)	Carbamazepine	Levetiracetam
	Sodium valproate	Clobazam
	Lamotrigine	Sodium valproate
	Oxcarbazepine	Lamotrigine
		Topiramate

avoided in women who may become pregnant. Carbamazepine is a potent enzyme inducer and may therefore interact with other medications, though oxcarbazepine may be an acceptable substitute.

It should be kept in mind that some AEDs should be avoided in the treatment of certain epilepsies as they can have a detrimental effect on seizure control. For the treatment of absence, atonic, tonic and myoclonic epilepsy, carbamazepine, gabapentin, vigabatrin, tiagabine, oxcarbazepine, pregabalin and phenytoin should be avoided. NICE (2012) also advises against using carbamazepine and oxcarbazepine in infantile spasms, myoclonic–astatic epilepsy and Landau–Kleffner, Lennox–Gastaut and Dravet syndromes.

Concerns remain about the toxicity of phenobarbitone and phenytoin and their impact on behaviour. This makes these medications unsuitable for the treatment of epilepsy in people with ID. Phenobarbitone and phenytoin should therefore only be used when attempts to replace them have failed or as a last resort.

Side effects of AEDs

People with ID are more prone to side effects than the general population; this can be related to their underlying brain pathology or to being on other medication for co-morbid psychiatric or medical problems and is partly why a slow titration is required.

Monitoring the side effects of AEDs in people with ID is a challenge, as patients do not usually volunteer such information due to their communication difficulties. Clinicians are advised to provide accessible information on the side effects of medication to patients and their carers and regularly monitor these with the help of other members of the MDT (e.g. nurses). Carers should be educated on how these side effects might present in someone with an ID, for example, as a change in behaviour such as self-injury, falls, aggression, not wanting to eat, etc.

It is vital to assess the temporal association of any behavioural change with the start or change of a medication. As a general rule, any new challenging behaviour that is out of character and temporally associated with use of a new medication (or a recent change in the dosage) could be a side effect (in the absence of other obvious causes such as infection or pain) until proven otherwise. Having said this, it is important not to attribute all behaviours or behaviours predating the initiation of the medications to side effects.

The *common side effects* caused by most AEDs include:
- Drowsiness
- Dizziness
- Ataxia
- Nausea and gastrointestinal disturbances
- Effect on speech
- Behaviour disturbances, including agitation, aggression and activation of psychosis (These side effects are generally dose related and respond to reduction in AED dose.)

In addition, individual medications have a range of *specific side effects*. For example, vigabatrin can cause visual field defects, and zonisamide and topiramate can cause weight loss and kidney stones (Table 4.11).

Table 4.11 Important side effects of AEDs.

AED	Side effects	Comments
Carbamazepine (Tegretol, Carbagen) + oxcarbazepine (Trileptal)	Blurred vision, dizziness, unsteadiness	Side effects are often dose related; reduced by using modified-release medications
	Mild transient generalised erythematous rash	Withdraw medication if this worsens or if other symptoms present
	Stevens–Johnson syndrome Blood dyscrasias: leucopenia, agranulocytosis, aplastic anaemia	Withdraw medication
	Induction of hepatic enzymes: Carbamazepine – potent inducer Oxcarbazepine – less potent induce	Lowers plasma concentration of: • Oral contraceptives • Sodium valproate • Ethosuximide • Clonazepam
	Hyponatraemia, oedema, disturbed bone metabolism	Reduced bone metabolism can cause osteomalacia
Ethosuximide (Zarontin, Emeside)	Gastrointestinal symptoms common, for example, nausea Hiccoughs Sedation, headache Significantly higher risk of acute psychiatric reactions following seizure control (forced normalisation) than with other anti-absence medications including sodium valproate	
Clobazam	Significant toxicity: sedation, dizziness, ataxia, diplopia	• Reported in 85% patients • Notable in 5–15% of them
	Tolerance to the anticonvulsant effect and withdrawal symptoms	
Clonazepam (Rivotril)	Drowsiness, ataxia, incoordination Behavioural and personality changes: hyperactivity, restlessness, short attention span, irritability, disruptiveness, aggressiveness Nystagmus, dizziness, hypotonia, blurred vision, diplopia, psychotic reaction Increased frequency of seizures and emergence of different types of seizures	
Gabapentin (Neurontin)	Drowsiness, fatigue, dizziness are common Increased frequency of seizures, especially deterioration of myoclonus Increased in behaviour problems, for example, hyperactivity, unprovoked outbursts of anger No idiosyncratic or hypersensitivity reactions or hepatotoxicity reported	
Lamotrigine (Lamictal)	Headache, diplopia, dizziness, ataxia and tremor are common Rash occurs in 3–5% of patients, necessitating withdrawal of medication Rarely Stevens–Johnson syndrome and erythema multiforme have been reported Low incidence of sedation	
Levetiracetam (Keppra)	Undue sedation, irritability and aggression in a small proportion of those who take it	
Pregabalin (Lyrica)	Somnolence, dizziness Weight gain, nausea	

(Continued)

Table 4.11 (*Continued*)

AED	Side effects	Comments
Topiramate (Topamax)	Somnolence, psychomotor slowing, speech disorder, nervousness	
	Dizziness, ataxia, nystagmus, parasthesiae	
	Emotional lability with mood disorders including depression	
	Altered behaviour, including psychotic symptoms	
	Hypersalivation, taste disorder	
	Adverse effect on cognition, for example, difficulty in word finding	
Sodium valproate (Epilim, Episenta, Convulex)	Weight gain (50% patients) often with nausea, vomiting, diarrhoea epigastric pain	
	Dizziness, drowsiness, sometimes postural tremor, nystagmus, rarely incoordination, ataxia	
	Idiosyncratic reactions, for example, hyperammonaemia, pancreatitis	
	Mild transient elevation of hepatic enzymes common; less common hepatotoxicity (may be dose related or idiosyncratic)	
	Altered behaviour, including psychotic symptoms	
	Anovulatory cycles, amenorrhoea and polycystic ovaries in women treated before age 20	
Tiagabine (Gabitril)	Dizziness and some central nervous system effects	
	Minimal adverse effect on cognition	
Zonisamide (Zonegran)	Nausea and diarrhoea	
	Anorexia and weight loss	
	Dizziness and drowsiness	
	Agitation	
	Withdraw if rash	

Of particular importance in people with ID is consideration of bone health. Many individuals have poor mobility and might be unable to exercise/follow a healthy diet and are therefore more at risk with AED treatment of developing negative bone metabolism.

Teratogenic effects of medication in women with ID of child-bearing age should be discussed in detail. It is often advisable to seek advice from other colleagues such as gynaecologists or paediatricians.

Illustrative case study 4.2

A 52-year-old man with Down syndrome and a recent diagnosis of Alzheimer's dementia developed unprovoked tonic–clonic seizures requiring admission to the accident and emergency department. He was put on sodium valproate, and the dose gradually increased over the next few weeks, which was effective in controlling the epilepsy. Unfortunately, he developed a severe tremor and daytime sedation, negatively affecting his quality of life. He was put on levetiracetam that was subsequently increased while tapering him gradually off his sodium valproate. This proved successful in managing his epilepsy with minimal side effects.

Antiepileptic polypharmacy

The refractory nature of seizures in many people with ID frequently results in the antiepileptic polypharmacy, often with only a marginal improvement in epilepsy control. For most people, it is unlikely that significant additional benefit will be achieved with more than two standard AEDs. Despite this, studies have shown that over 40% of patient received two or more AEDs. In addition, up to a quarter of those on AEDs are on concurrent antipsychotics, which may affect the seizure frequency.

Orphan antiepileptics

These are medications only licensed for use in specific syndromes. For example, add-on stiripentol is currently being used in treating epilepsy in Dravet syndrome (severe myoclonic epilepsy of infancy). Similarly, rufinamide is licensed as an add-on treatment for intractable epilepsy in people with a diagnosis of Lennox–Gastaut syndrome.

Newer antiepileptics

Lacosamide (Vimpat) acts via sodium channels and is licensed as an add-on AED for treatment of focal epilepsy with or without secondary generalisation. It has also been shown to be an effective analgesic in people with diabetic neuropathy. It can cause similar dose-related side effects as other AEDs (e.g. dizziness), alongside specific side effects such as first-degree heart block (P–R interval prolongation).

Eslicarbazepine acetate (Zebinix) acts in a similar fashion to oxcarbazepine and has a better side effect profile than carbamazepine.

Retigabine (Trobalt) is licensed as an add-on for treatment of focal epilepsy with or without secondary generalisation. It acts on potassium channels and might also be used for neuropathic pain and migraine but can cause blue discoloration of the skin, pigment changes in the retina, QT interval prolongation and psychiatric side effects.

Perampanel (Fycompa) acts on AMPA receptors and is licensed for treatment of refractory partial seizures. In addition to common side effects similar to other AEDs, it might increase the risk of psychiatric/behavioural disorders.

Therapeutic medication monitoring

NICE has examined the evidence regarding therapeutic medication monitoring of AEDs and concluded that routine monitoring of AED blood levels does not improve seizure control. Therefore, levels should only be checked if clinically indicated. Such indications include:

- Detection/suspicion of non-adherence to the prescribed AED
- Suspected toxicity of the AED
- Adjustment of dose, specifically in the case of phenytoin
- Management of pharmacokinetic interactions

Interactions between AEDs

Table 4.12 describes commonly encountered and known significant interactions between AEDs.

Table 4.12 Significant interactions known to occur between antiepileptics.

Medications causing interaction	Medications affected by interaction												
	CBZ	CLB	CLN	ESM	GBP	LTG	LEV	PB	PHT	PRM	TGB	TOP	VPA
Carbamazepine (CBZ)		NE	↓CLN	↓ESM	NE	↓LTG	NE	↑↓PB	↑↓PHT	↓PRM	↓TGB	↓TOP	↓VPA
Clobazam (CLB)	NE		NE	NE	NE	NE	NE	NE	NE	NE	NE	NE	↑VPA
Clonazepam (CLN)	↓CBZ	NE		NE	NE	NE	NE	NE	↑↓PHT	NE	NE	NE	NE
Ethosuximide (ESM)	NE	NE	NE		NE	NE	NE	NE	NE	NE	NE	NE	NE
Gabapentin (GBP)	NE	NE	NE	NE		NE	NE	NE	NE	NE	NE	NE	NE
Lamotrigine (LTG)	↑CBZ	NE	NE	NE	NE		NE	NE	NE	NE	NE	NE	NE
Levetiracetam (LEV)	NE	NE	NE	NE	NE	NE		NE	NE	NE	NE	NE	NE
Phenobarbitone (PB)	↓CBZ	NE	↓CLN	↓ESM	NE	↓LTG	NE		↓PHT	NE	↓TGB	↓TOP	↓VPA
Phenytoin (PHT)	↓CBZ	NE	NE	↓ESM	NE	↓LTG	NE	↓↑PB		NE	↓TGB	↓TOP	↓VPA
Primidone (PRM)	↓CBZ	NE	↓CLN	↓ESM	NE	↓LTG	NE	NE	↓↑PHT		↓TGB	↓TOP	↓VPA
Tiagabine (TGB)	NE	NE	NE	NE	NE	NE	NE	NE	NE	NE		NE	NE
Topiramate (TOP)	NE	NE	NE	NE	NE	NE	NE	NE	NE	NE	NE		NE
Sodium valproate (VPA)	↑CBZ	NE	NE	↑ESM	NE	↑LTG	NE	↑PB	↑↓PHT	NE	NE	NE	

NE, no interaction expected (in most cases).

↑, increased medication level of specified medication.

↓, decreased medication level of specified medication.

↑↓, increased or decreased in level of specified medication.

Prolonged or repeated seizures

Any individual who has generalised tonic–clonic seizures lasting for 5 minutes or more or three or more seizures in an hour should receive urgent treatment, usually with the administration of rectal diazepam or buccal midazolam. For most adults, a dose of 10–20 mg is recommended. In some cases, this can be repeated after 10 minutes; however, the potential for respiratory depression must be taken into account.

More recently, the administration of buccal midazolam has become popular as it can be more socially acceptable and easier to administer than rectal diazepam. For some children's services in ID, it has become the medication of choice. Buccal midazolam should be administered by trained clinical personnel. It can be administered by family members or carers if they have undergone the appropriate training and there is a previously agreed protocol in place from the specialist team.

Refractory epilepsy

When there are ongoing seizures despite optimal medication therapy, this is termed refractory epilepsy. In the general population, approximately 20–30% of people with active epilepsy suffer from refractory epilepsy. The incidence is higher in those with ID.

Refractoriness of seizures varies according to the underlying and concomitant conditions. For example, a 12-year follow-up study of ID patients with epilepsy showed that 79% without abnormal neurology became seizure-free (the same proportion as the general population), compared to only 39% of those with abnormal neurology. Individuals with cerebral palsy often have an early onset of seizures that are difficult to control.

NICE recommends that combination therapy (adjunctive or 'add-on' therapy) should only be considered when attempts at monotherapy with AEDs have not resulted in seizure freedom. If trials of combination therapy do not bring about worthwhile benefits, treatment should revert to the regimen (monotherapy or combination therapy) that has proved most acceptable to the patient in terms of providing the best balance between effectiveness in reducing seizure frequency and tolerability of side effects.

Neurosurgery

Neurosurgery is a final option for those with severe refractory seizures. There are various different procedures including focal resections, temporal lobectomy, multilobar resections and hemispherectomy. It also includes functional procedures such as multiple subpial transection, vagal nerve stimulation (VNS) and corpus callosectomy. A diagnosis of ID should not be considered a contraindication to using surgery or VNS.

In patients with cerebral dysgenesis and severe drop attacks, procedures such as focal resection, hemispherectomy and corpus callosotomy may prove beneficial. VNS may be particularly helpful for intractable cases where there is a good seizure warning, such that the device can be activated at these times to halt seizure progression.

A substantial proportion of patients with ID improve following surgery, and some become totally seizure-free. However, the risk–benefit ratio of surgery must be assessed on an individual basis. When considering a referral for neurosurgery, the following factors should be included:
• The aetiology of the epilepsy and the ID
• Other co-morbidities
• The investigations that have been undergone prior to surgery, which should include neurophysiological and neuropsychological testing as well as neuroimaging
• The support services available to this client group.

Psychosocial input

When managing epilepsy in the ID population, it is important to consider psychosocial aspects of care and assessment alongside pharmacological or biological treatments. For example, starting an antiepileptic is not enough if a significant environmental risk is missed (which would be screened by a risk assessment from occupational therapy).

Social services are an important part of the MDT for epilepsy management. They can provide necessary adaptions including assisted technology, such as epilepsy bed sensors to alert a carer that a patient requires urgent help. As part of the MDT, they can also make assessments regarding benefits, respite facilities, day centres/day activities, training, voluntary/supported employment and residential and supported living placement that the patient is entitled to. They can also carry out a carer's need assessment, which all carers and families are entitled to.

Patient information

As well as keeping up to date with epilepsy management, it is important that the clinician takes an active role in educating patients, family members and carers, at the appropriate level.

Patients and carers should be provided with accessible information (either through leaflets or websites) and be offered training on epilepsy. Information on SUDEP should be included as well as how to deal with emergency situations (including the safe use of epilepsy rescue medication) (Table 4.13).

Table 4.13 Useful patient information websites.

www.epilepsy.org.uk
www.epilepsyresearch.org.uk
www.epilepsysociety.org.uk
www.sudep.org
www.sudepaware.org

Discussion case study 4.3

A 44-year-old lady with autism and generalised epilepsy who lives in a supported living accommodation is seen in your clinic for a review of her epilepsy control. You notice that over the past two years, her lamotrigine has been gradually increased by your trainee doctors to a maximum of 125 mg bid with no success in controlling her tonic–clonic seizures.

On further history taking, you realise that she self-administers her medication but has not let her support workers in to monitor the administration of medication. Further observation by staff, who finally manage to get into her flat, reveals that she has hoarded her medication over the past 12 months. You arrange for another review but notice that she becomes extremely anxious when you discuss compliance with treatment. She also appears confused when you discuss side effects and struggles to repeat what you have just explained to her in spite of appearing fluent superficially.

• What are the main issues in the management of her epilepsy?
• What are the non-pharmacological aspects of treating her epilepsy?
• Who else would you involve in your management plan?
• What are the risks in this case?

References

Commission on Classification and Terminology of the International League Against Epilepsy (1981) Proposal for revised clinical and electrographic classification of epileptic seizures. *Epilepsia* 22:489–501.

National Institute for Health and Care Excellence (2012) The epilepsies. The diagnosis and management of the epilepsies in adult and children in primary and secondary care. Clinical guidelines CG137 Available at: http://guidance.nice.org.uk/CG137 (accessed 6 January 2015).

Trimble MR, Schmitz B (eds.) (2011) *The Neuropsychiatry of Epilepsy*. Cambridge University Press, New York.

Further reading

Alarcon G, Nashef L, Cross H, et al. (2009) *Epilepsy*. Oxford Specialist Handbooks in Neurology. Oxford University Press, New York.

Amiet C, Gourfinkel-An I, Bouzamondo A, et al. (2008) Epilepsy in autism is associated with intellectual disability and gender: evidence from a meta-analysis. *Biol Psychiatry* 64(7):577–82.

Betts T (1998) *Epilepsy, Psychiatry and Learning Difficulty*. Martin Dunitz and Parthenon Publishing, London.

Branford D, Bhaumik S, Duncan F (1998) Epilepsy in adults with learning disabilities. *Seizure* 6:473–7.

Brodie MJ, Schachter SC, Kwam P (2009) *Fast Facts: Epilepsy*. 4th edn. Health Press Ltd., Oxford.

Chapman M, Iddon P, Atkinson K, et al. (2011) The misdiagnosis of epilepsy in people with intellectual disabilities: a systematic review. *Seizure* 20(2):101–6.

Corbett J (1981) Epilepsy and mental retardation. In: Reyonds ER, Trimble MR (eds.) *Epilepsy and Psychiatry*. Churchill Livingstone, Edinburgh: pp. 138–46.

Deb S (2007) Epilepsy in people with mental retardation. In: Jacobson JW, Mulick JA (eds.) *Handbook of Mental Retardation and Developmental Disabilities*. Kluwer Academic Publishers, New York: pp. 81–96.

Forsgren L, Edvinsson SO, Blomquist HK, et al. (1990) Epilepsy in a population of mentally retarded children and adults. *Epilepsy Res* 6:234–8.

George JR, Davis GG (1998) Comparison of anti-epileptic drug levels in different cases of sudden death. *J Forensic Sci* 43:598–603.

Goulden J, Shinnar S, Koller H, et al. (1991) Epilepsy in children with mental retardation: a cohort study. *Epilepsia* 32:690–7.

Kerr MP, Mensah S, Besag F, et al. (2011) International consensus clinical practice statements for the treatment of neuropsychiatric conditions associated with epilepsy. International League of Epilepsy (ILAE) Commission on the Neuropsychiatric Aspects of Epilepsy. *Epilepsia* 52(11):2133–8.

Kiani R, Tyrer F, Jesu A, et al. (2013) Mortality from sudden unexpected death in epilepsy (SUDEP) in a cohort of adults with intellectual disability. *J Intellect Disabil Res* 58(6):508–20.

Kirkham F (1995) Epilepsy and mental retardation. In: Hopkins A, Shorvon S, Cascmo G (eds.) *Epilepsy*. Chapman & Hall Medical, London: pp. 503–520.

McGrother C, Bhaumik S, Thorp C, et al. (2006) Epilepsy in adults with intellectual disabilities: prevalence, associations and service implications. *Seizure* 15(6):376–86.

McVicker R, Shanks OEP, McClelland R (1994) Prevalence and associated features of epilepsy in adults with Down's syndrome. *Br J Psychiatry* 164:528–32.

Nashef L, Fish DR, Gamer S, et al. (1995) Sudden death in epilepsy — a study of incidence in a young cohort with epilepsy and learning difficulty. *Epilepsia* 36:1187–94.

Olsson I, Steffenburg S, Gillberg C (1988) Epilepsy in autism and autistic-like conditions. A population-based study. *Arch Neurol* 45:666–8.

Ring H, Zia A, Bateman N, et al. (2009) How is epilepsy treated in people with a learning disability? A retrospective observational study of 183 individuals. *Seizure* 18(4):264–8.

Steffenburg U, Hagberg G, Kyllerman M (1996) Characteristics of seizures in a population-based series of mentally retarded children with active epilepsy. *Epilepsia* 39(9):850–6.

CHAPTER 5

Dementia in People with Intellectual Disability

Satheesh Kumar Gangadharan & Amala Jovia Maria Jesu

Leicestershire Partnership NHS Trust, Leicester, UK

> Those with dementia are still people and they still have stories and they still have character and they're all individuals and they're all unique. And they just need to be interacted with on a human level.
>
> *Carey Mulligan*

Definition

Dementia is a clinical syndrome of acquired cognitive impairment produced by brain dysfunction. It is associated with deterioration in memory, thinking, behaviour and the ability to perform everyday activities. Although it is often seen in older people, it is neither an inevitable part of normal ageing process, nor is it a problem of elderly exclusively. Dementia has a significant impact on carers, family and general society.

Prevalence

People with intellectual disabilities (ID) have a higher risk of developing dementia when compared to the general population. Studies investigating the rates of clinical dementia in people with ID have reported variable prevalence rates depending on the diagnostic criteria used. In a study by Strydom et al. (2007) using DSM-IV criteria, prevalence rates for clinical dementia in ID were observed to be 13.1% in those over 60 years and 18.3% in those 65 years and over.

The Frith Prescribing Guidelines for People with Intellectual Disability, Third Edition.
Edited by Sabyasachi Bhaumik, David Branford, Mary Barrett and Satheesh Kumar Gangadharan.
© 2015 John Wiley & Sons, Ltd. Published 2015 by John Wiley & Sons, Ltd.

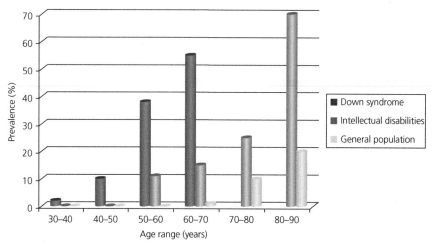

Figure 5.1 Age-related prevalence rates of dementia in Down syndrome, in intellectual disabilities excluding Down syndrome and in general population.

Down syndrome, the most frequent known cause of ID, is associated with an even higher risk of developing dementia particularly dementia of Alzheimer's type. Prevalence of clinical dementia in people with Down syndrome starts at less than 5% in the 30–39-year age group increasing dramatically to 50% in over 50s and up to 75% in people over the age of 60 years. The peak incidence is believed to be in the early 50s.

In people with ID without Down syndrome, the age of onset is brought forwards slightly, along with a higher prevalence rate compared to general population. The cause for this higher prevalence rate is unknown due to lack of valid studies in this population. This group has a similar range of causes of dementia as the general population. The four most common causes of dementia are Alzheimer's disease, Lewy body dementia, vascular dementia and fronto-temporal dementia (Figure 5.1).

Clinical presentation

The common presentation of dementia in people with ID includes memory loss and deterioration in speech, personality and behavioural changes, disorientation and functional deterioration (Table 5.1). A significant proportion present with seizures or incontinence, which are seen only in later stages of dementia in people without ID. Frontal lobe symptoms such as slowness in activities and speech, loss of interest, withdrawal and emotional and behaviour problems may also be the presenting symptoms of dementia in people with ID.

Table 5.1 Main features of dementia.

Cognitive	Decline in memory, aphasia, apraxia, agnosia, executive dysfunction
Non-cognitive	Emotional lability, irritability, apathy, coarsening of social behaviour
Social	Decline in self-care and daily living skills
	Interpersonal difficulties and behaviour problems

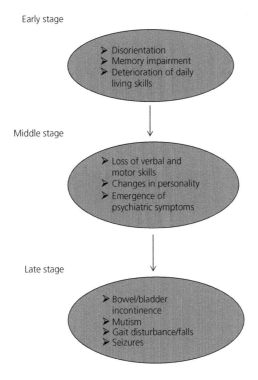

Figure 5.2 Clinical stages of dementia in people with ID.

Clinical stages of dementia in people with ID

It is difficult to identify the stages of dementia in people with ID due to the variability in presentation as well as variability in the level of premorbid cognitive and adaptive skills. Figure 5.2 gives a general guideline in identifying the early, middle and late stages of dementia in people with ID.

Diagnosis of dementia in people with ID

The diagnosis of dementia requires evidence of a definitive change in cognitive functioning such as impairment in memory, language ability (aphasia), ability to perform complex tasks (apraxia) and orientation in time and place. These are associated with changes in daily living skills, behaviour and personality (DSM-IV, ICD-10).

The objective measurement of cognitive function and the detection of any changes in people with moderate or severe ID remain a challenge for clinicians.

ASSESSMENT CHALLENGES

- Difficulty for the person in providing a subjective account due to diminished ability to think abstractly and to communicate
- Difficulties in recognising subtle clinical changes due to variable level of pre-existing impairment in cognitive functions and adaptive skills
- Presence of other disabilities such as sensory impairments and autism masking or altering the presentation
- Difficulties in co-operating with investigations such as blood tests, sensory screening and neuroimaging

A number of clinical problems may mimic dementia in those with Down syndrome. These disorders may also coexist with dementia and require treatment. Table 5.2 gives a list of other possible causes of dementia-like symptoms to consider before making a diagnosis of dementia.

Table 5.2 Other conditions which mimic or overlap symptoms of dementia.

Causation	Details
Psychosocial	Bereavement, loss of contact with key individuals, changes in day activities, any significant stressful life events (e.g. sexual or physical abuse), etc.
Environment	Increased demand from a new environment, lack of adequate stimulation in the environment
Sensory impairments	Hearing deficits, visual impairment (cataracts), etc.
Epilepsy	Onset of seizures or increase in seizures
Pain	Abdominal pain, backache, discomfort from severe constipation, etc.
Metabolic changes	Hypothyroidism, anaemia, vitamin B_{12} or folate deficiencies, hypo- or hyperglycaemia, electrolyte disturbances, etc.
Other brain conditions	Haematoma, infections affecting brain as well as brain tumours
Mental health conditions	Depression, psychotic conditions, severe forms of anxiety, etc.
Medication	Raised levels of anti-epileptic medications, medications with cholinergic side effects, multiple medications, etc.

Assessment

The National Task Group on Intellectual Disabilities and Dementia Practices (Mayo Clinic Proceedings 2013) recommends a nine-step approach. A detailed description of the assessment process is also provided in the Royal College report CR155. Table 5.3 has used information from both sources.

Table 5.3 Key points for the assessment of dementia in people with ID.

Relevant assessment	Details
Medical history, psychiatric history and psychosocial history	Medical history to include cardiovascular history, presence of any neurological conditions, history of head injury, evidence of metabolic disorders such as hypothyroidism (including if it is adequately treated if already diagnosed)
	Psychiatric history to include any evidence of depression either at present or in the past, presence of bipolar disorder or any psychotic condition
	Bereavement, changes in social relationships, presence of any stressful events, etc.
Historical description of baseline functioning	Where possible collected using a structured tool covering all areas of functioning
Picture of current functioning	An informant questionnaire should be used to gather the information systematically. Please see the list of instruments available for this purpose (Appendix 5.1)
Review of medications	A thorough review of medications with a particular focus on newly added medication or changes in the dose. The following medications have a higher risk of causing cognitive impairment: psychoactive, anti-epileptic or cholinergic and those with sedating properties
Family history	Family history of early-onset dementia, cardiovascular conditions, stroke, diabetes, rheumatoid arthritis, SLE, etc.
Environment	Quality of physical environment, mix of people with intellectual disabilities in the residential settings, quality and quantity of day activities
	Staffing levels, staff characteristics: attitudes and competence, etc.
Physical examination	A thorough physical examination where possible, physical health screening where a physical examination is not possible (e.g. OK physical health check)
Investigations	Full blood count, urea and electrolytes, blood sugar, thyroid function, liver function, B_{12} and folate level, lipid profile, sensory screening, electrocardiograph (ECG), MRI brain scan or CT head if practical
Mental state examination and cognitive assessment	A number of structured tools are available to aid the cognitive assessment in people with ID (Appendix 5.2)
Synthesis of information and formulation	Assessments are often undertaken by a number of professionals and therefore information collected by all should be discussed to formulate and make a clear diagnosis

Illustrative case study 5.1

> Peter is a 55-year-old gentleman with mild ID of unknown aetiology who lives with his parents. He has been reasonably independent until recently. He had been able to look after his personal care with occasional reminders and minimal supervision from his parents. Peter had always helped his parents around the home, as well as cleaning the patio and helping his father in doing gardening. He attends a day centre where he did voluntary work. He was previously able to go to the nearby town on his own and do some limited shopping as well. He is able to communicate well although he can at times struggle to understand the meaning of some words. He has limited reading and writing skills.
>
> Peter presented with forgetfulness and occasional confusion (not knowing where he is, not being able to remember the task he is supposed to do, etc.). In this case, the presentation is somewhat similar to that in those without ID; a detailed cognitive assessment was possible, although Peter needed support and some adaptation of the method. He was able to co-operate with a full physical examination and investigations leading to the diagnosis of a dementia of Alzheimer's type.

Illustrative case study 5.2

> Mary is 45 and has Down syndrome and moderate ID. She lives in supported living and attends a day centre. She needs support from carers for her personal care and cannot travel independently. Mary had a vocabulary of 50 words and can use some limited Makaton signs but cannot read or write. She presented with a change in behaviour that included being noisy and disruptive in group sessions, not sleeping well at night as well as refusing to accept support for personal care. Once or twice, she has lashed out at the carers who were trying to provide personal care. A careful history taking by the psychiatrist showed that there has been subtle changes in her skills (ability to put on her dress with her often doing it in the wrong way around, ability to follow instructions in the group sessions, ability to engage in a task for a period of time, etc.). A contributory factor was that there had been a number of changes in her care staff over the last few months. Unfortunately, there was no clear record of her premorbid skills: she moved into the supported living after her mother died about 2 years back and had not previously had input from health services. Assessment found no evidence of depression or other mental health problems.
>
> Mary would not co-operate with a full physical examination, and therefore, an 'OK physical health check' was undertaken by the community ID nurse. It showed that Mary was having some difficulty in hearing as well as constantly pinching her ears. Apart from the ear problem, health screening has not shown any evidence of physical health problems. Mary would not co-operate with MRI or CT scans.
>
> After desensitisation work by the community nurse, the GP was able to examine Mary's ears and take blood samples. Ear examination showed wax impaction, which was successfully treated using warm olive oil. This improved her behaviour to some extent (stopped pinching the ears and was able to follow instructions better than before), but she continued to have the other changes described earlier. Blood testing did not reveal any abnormal findings.
>
> Using the Dementia Questionnaire for People with Learning Disabilities (DLD), a community nurse gathered Mary's level of adaptive skills at the point of original assessment and repeated this after 6 months. Analysis of the two DLD scores revealed that Mary's cognitive and social scores increased over a 6-month period, indicating increase in impairment over this period. Over the 6-month period, Mary also started becoming

incontinent, slightly unsteady while walking and unable to feed herself neatly as she used to do. An occupational therapist also completed an assessment of Mary's motor and processing skills, which highlighted problems not previously observed.

A diagnosis of dementia was made by the psychiatrist after analysing the information gathered.

Table 5.4 Evidence base for medication treatment in dementia.

Medications for cognitive symptoms of dementia	Overview of evidence from specific medicine trials of benefits in dementia
Acetylcholinesterase (AChE) inhibitors: 　Donepezil 　Galantamine 　Rivastigmine	The three AChE inhibitors donepezil, galantamine and rivastigmine are recommended as options for managing mild to moderate Alzheimer's disease (National Institute for Health and Care Excellence, 2011) • Evidence in people with ID and dementia is limited • Prasher et al. (2005): People who were treated with rivastigmine had less decline over 24 weeks in global functioning and adaptive behaviours • Prasher et al. (2002): Double-blind placebo-controlled trial of donepezil showed that the improvement at 24 weeks was statistically non-significant. The sample size of the study was too small to explore the efficacy in the subgroups of mild to moderate disease • Lott et al. (2002): In their open-label study on donepezil, they found that treatment resulted in significant improvement in scores on the Down Syndrome Dementia Scale (Gedye, 1995). However, there were methodological drawbacks • Prasher et al. (2003): In their open-label study on donepezil treatment for people with Down's syndrome, they found that treatment with the anti-dementia medication was associated with initial improvement in global functioning and adaptive behaviours. Follow-up at 104 weeks found that while there was deterioration in both treatment and control groups, it was significantly less in the treatment group • Prasher et al (2013): Both oral and transdermal rivastigmine treatments were associated with significantly less decline in both cognitive and global functioning over a 6-month period compared to people on no treatment
NMDA antagonist Memantine	Memantine is recommended as an option for managing Alzheimer's disease for people with moderate Alzheimer's disease who have non-cognitive symptoms and/or behaviour that challenges and are intolerant of or have a contraindication to AChE inhibitors, as well as people with severe Alzheimer's disease (National Institute for Health and Care Excellence, 2011) A prospective randomised double-blind controlled trial comparing memantine with placebo in people with Down syndrome did not find any significant difference. However, this study used patients with Down syndrome with and without clinical diagnosis of dementia and therefore limits the scope of clinical implication

Management of dementia

Medications only have a limited role in the management of dementia. Detailed guidance on the management of dementia in people with ID is available in the Faculty of Intellectual Disability of the Royal College of Psychiatrists document (CR155); however, the key principles in the use of medications for dementia in people with ID are summarised in Table 5.4.

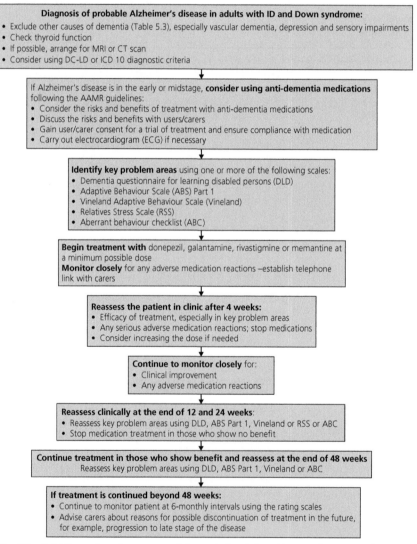

Diagnosis of probable Alzheimer's disease in adults with ID and Down syndrome:
- Exclude other causes of dementia (Table 5.3), especially vascular dementia, depression and sensory impairments
- Check thyroid function
- If possible, arrange for MRI or CT scan
- Consider using DC-LD or ICD 10 diagnostic criteria

If Alzheimer's disease is in the early or midstage, **consider using anti-dementia medications** following the AAMR guidelines:
- Consider the risks and benefits of treatment with anti-dementia medications
- Discuss the risks and benefits with users/carers
- Gain user/carer consent for a trial of treatment and ensure compliance with medication
- Carry out electrocardiogram (ECG) if necessary

Identify key problem areas using one or more of the following scales:
- Dementia questionnaire for learning disabled persons (DLD)
- Adaptive Behaviour Scale (ABS) Part 1
- Vineland Adaptive Behaviour Scale (Vineland)
- Relatives Stress Scale (RSS)
- Aberrant behaviour checklist (ABC)

Begin treatment with donepezil, galantamine, rivastigmine or memantine at a minimum possible dose
Monitor closely for any adverse medication reactions –establish telephone link with carers

Reassess the patient in clinic after 4 weeks:
- Efficacy of treatment, especially in key problem areas
- Any serious adverse medication reactions; stop medications
- Consider increasing the dose if needed

Continue to monitor closely for:
- Clinical improvement
- Any adverse medication reactions

Reassess clinically at the end of 12 and 24 weeks:
- Reassess key problem areas using DLD, ABS Part 1, Vineland or RSS or ABC
- Stop medication treatment in those who show no benefit

Continue treatment in those who show benefit and reassess at the end of 48 weeks
Reassess key problem areas using DLD, ABS Part 1, Vineland or ABC

If treatment is continued beyond 48 weeks:
- Continue to monitor patient at 6-monthly intervals using the rating scales
- Advise carers about reasons for possible discontinuation of treatment in the future, for example, progression to late stage of the disease

Algorithm 5.1 Diagnosis and treatment of dementia in adults with ID and Down syndrome.

Pharmacological interventions for the cognitive symptoms of dementia

A number of medications are used in delaying the progress of dementia as in general population. Evidence base for the use of medication in people with ID is currently limited.

Algorithm 5.1 provides guidance for the use of anti-dementia medication in people with ID.

Table 5.5 Pharmacological interventions for behavioural and psychological symptoms of dementia (BPSD): the table summarises the evidence from non-ID population.

Medications for BPSD	Overview of evidence base
Antipsychotics	Second-generation antipsychotics (SGA) were once widely recommended in dementia-related behaviour disturbance, but their use now is highly controversial. Three reasons for this are (i) small effect size, (ii) poor tolerability and (iii) tentative association with increased mortality
	Evidence from non-ID population demonstrated minor effectiveness advantages for olanzapine and risperidone over placebo, but all medications were poorly tolerated due to sedation, confusion and EPSEs
	In the UK and the USA, warnings have been issued regarding increased mortality with olanzapine, risperidone, quetiapine and aripiprazole when used in dementia due to an association with stroke
	Amisulpride has been used, but its safety in this group of patients is unknown. Traditional antipsychotic medications like sulpiride have also been used although sedation and anticholinergic effects can cause deterioration of cognitive impairment
Acetylcholinesterase inhibitors and memantine	National Institute for Health and Care Excellence, 2011 recommends that people with mild to moderate Alzheimer's disease who have non-cognitive symptoms may be offered an acetylcholinesterase inhibitor if a non-pharmacological approach is inappropriate or has been ineffective and antipsychotic medications are inappropriate or have been ineffective
	People with moderate to severe Alzheimer's disease who are intolerant of or have a contraindication to acetylcholinesterase inhibitors may be offered memantine
Antidepressants	To treat symptoms of depression, selective serotonin reuptake inhibitors (SSRIs) are preferred, but attention is needed to the risk of developing low sodium levels. Sertraline has some evidence for its effectiveness in the treatment of depression in dementia
	There is emerging evidence that SSRIs may be used for treatment of agitation in dementia. Many clinicians prefer trazodone for which also there is some evidence available
Mood stabilisers	Medications such as carbamazepine or sodium valproate may be considered if there is evidence of rapid cycling mood disorder or significant mood fluctuations

There is currently no evidence for the use of these medications in people with ID and dementia.

Treatment of behavioural and psychological symptoms of dementia

Psychotropic medications have only a limited role in the management of neuropsychiatric symptoms in people with ID and dementia. They should only be considered if:

• Other environmental/psychosocial approaches have had limited or no benefit.

• The risk from the symptoms is assessed as high.

Use of these medications should only be considered after a very careful evaluation of the risks and benefits in each individual circumstance (Table 5.5).

THE BELOW PRINCIPLES SHOULD BE FOLLOWED:

> • The risks and benefits should be shared with the individual (if the individual is able to understand the information) and carers. In particular, cerebrovascular risk factors should be assessed, and the possible increased risk of stroke/transient ischaemic attack and possible adverse effects on cognition discussed.
> • Target symptoms are identified and monitored regularly.
> • Changes in cognition should be assessed and recorded at regular intervals.
> • Alternative medication should be considered if necessary.
> • Medication should be started at the lowest possible dose and titrated slowly. Only the lowest effective dose of the medication should be continued.
> • Treatment should be time limited and regularly reviewed (every 3 months or according to clinical need).

Discussion case study 5.3

> Brenda is a 55-year-old lady with Down syndrome living in a residential home. Carers report deterioration in her personal hygiene, which they attribute to loss of personal care skills. She tends to lose her way around the home. She is often forgetful and accuses other residents of stealing her things. According to care staff, these changes have been noted since the demise of her mother 6 months ago, at which point she came to live at this home. She has poor sleep at night and has been found by carers on occasions in the back garden appearing confused. She has mild LD and not previously known to services. She has now been referred by the GP for further assessment.
> Questions:
> • How will you assess this case?
> • What are the diagnostic possibilities?
> • What will be the management plan?

References

Haxby, J.V. (1989) Neuropsychological evaluation of adults with Down syndrome: patterns of selective impairment in non-demented old adults. *Journal of Mental Deficiency Research*, 33 (Pt. 3), 193–210.

Moran, J.A., Rafii, M.S., Keller, S.M., Singh, B.K. & Janicki, M.P. (2013) The National Task Group on intellectual disabilities and dementia practices consensus recommendations for the evaluation and management of dementia in adults with intellectual disabilities. *Mayo Clinic Proceedings*, 88 (8), 831–840.

National Institute for Health and Care Excellence (2011, March) Donepezil, galantamine, rivastigmine and memantine for the treatment of Alzheimer's disease. NICE technology appraisals (TA217). http://www.nice.org.uk/guidance/ta217 (accessed 6 January 2015).

Strydom, A., Livingston, G., King, M. & Hassiotis, A. (2007) Prevalence of dementia in intellectual disability using different diagnostic criteria. *British Journal of Pharmacology*, 191, 150–157.

Further reading

Cooper, S-A. (1997) High prevalence of dementia amongst people with learning disabilities not attributed to Down's syndrome. *Psychological Medicine*, 27, 609–616.

Deb, S. (2003) Dementia in people with an intellectual disability. *Reviews in Clinical Gerontology*, 13, 137–144.

Holland, A.J., Hon, J., Huppert, F., Stevens, F. & Watson, P. (1998) Population-based study of the prevalence and presentation of dementia in adults with Down's syndrome. *British Journal of Psychiatry*, 172, 493–498.

The British Psychological Society and the Royal College of Psychiatrists (2009) *Dementia and People with Learning Disabilities; Guidance on the Assessment, Diagnosis, Treatment and Support of People with Learning Disabilities Who Develop Dementia.* Leicester: British Psychological Society.

Evidence base references

Lott, I.T., Osann, K., Doran, E. & Nelson, L. (2002) Down syndrome and Alzheimer's disease: response to Donepezil. *Archives of Neurology*, 59, 1133–1136.

Prasher, V.P., Huxley, A. & Haque, M.S. (2002) A 24 week, double blind, placebo controlled trial of donepezil in patients with Down syndrome and Alzheimer's disease – pilot study. *International Journal of Geriatric Psychiatry*, 17, 270–278.

Prasher, V.P., Adams, C. & Holder, R. (2003) Long term safety and efficacy of donepezil in the treatment of dementia in Alzheimer's disease in adults with Down syndrome: open label study. *International Journal of Geriatric Psychiatry*, 8, 549–551.

Prasher, V.P., Fung, N. & Adams, C. (2005) Rivastigmine in the treatment of dementia in adults with Down syndrome. *International Journal of Geriatric Psychiatry*, 20, 496–497.

Prasher, V.P., Sachdeva, N., Adams, C. & Haque, M.S. (2013) Rivastigmine transdermal patches in the treatment of dementia in Alzheimer's disease in adults with Down syndrome – pilot study. *International Journal of Geriatric Psychiatry*, 28, 219–220.

References for questionnaires

Albert, M. & Cohen, C. (1992) The Test for Severe Impairment: an instrument for the assessment of people with severe cognitive dysfunction. *Journal of the American Geriatric Society*, 40, 449–453.

Ball, S., Holland, T., Huppert, F.A., Treppner, P. & Dodd, K. (2006) *CAMDEX-DS: The Cambridge Examination for Mental Disorders of Older People with Down's Syndrome and Others with Intellectual Disabilities*. Cambridge, UK: Cambridge University Press.

Evenhuis, H.M. (1996) Further evaluation of the Dementia questionnaire for persons with mental retardation. *Journal of Intellectual Disability Research*, 40, 369–373.

Gedye, A. (1995) *Dementia Scale for Down's Syndrome – Manual*. Vancouver: Gedye Research & Consulting.

Sparrow, S.S., Cichetti, D.V. & Balla, D.A. (2007) *Vineland II: Vineland Adaptive Behaviour Scales* (2nd ed.). Oxford: Pearson.

Sturmey, P., Tsiouris, J.A. & Patti, P. (2003) The psychometric properties of the Multi-Dimensional Observation Scale for Elderly Subjects (MOSES) in middle aged and older populations of people with mental retardation. *International Journal of Geriatric Psychiatry*, 18, 131–134.

Appendix 5.1 Tools for screening dementia in ID

Questionnaire	Useful information
Dementia Questionnaire for People with Learning Disabilities (DLD) (Evenhuis 1996)	It has 50 items and 8 subscales. Carers can complete this questionnaire by themselves. It takes approximately 15–20 minutes to complete. Cognitive and non-cognitive scores can be summed up separately. A diagnosis for dementia is considered if the sum of cognitive scores increases by 9 points or the total score increases by 13
Down Syndrome Dementia Scale (DSDS) (Gedye 1995)	There are 60 questions and these are divided up between early, middle and late stages of dementia. This is the only instrument that attempts to identify the stages of dementia. It requires a trained person, that is, a psychologist to administer, and ideally, two informants should be interviewed
Multidimensional Observation Scale for Elderly Subjects (MOSES) (Sturmey et al. 2003)	It is a 40-item questionnaire covering five areas – self-help skills, disorientation, depression, irritability and social withdrawal. An informant makes the rating based on one week of direct observation, and it can be completed in 10–15 minutes
Daily Living Skills Questionnaire (DLSQ) (National Institute for Ageing 1989)	This is a 28-item test assessing the competency in areas of daily living skills. It covers dressing (5 items), manual dexterity (2 items), eating (6 items), personal hygiene (5 items), housekeeping (5 items) and orientation (5 items)
Vineland Adaptive Behaviour Scale (Sparrow et al. 1984)	This is not specific for dementia but very useful in identifying changes in adaptive behaviour

Appendix 5.2 Neuro psychological tests for the diagnosis of dementia in ID

Instrument	Useful information
Down Syndrome Mental State Examination (DSMSE) (Haxby 1989)	This consists of a battery of neuropsychological tests assessing a broad range of skills including recall of personal information, orientation to seasons and day of the week, memory, language, visuospatial function and praxis. A verbal response is required for most of the tests
Tests for Severe Impairment (TSI) (Albert and Cohen 1992)	This was originally developed to measure cognitive impairment in people with severe dementia. The six domains included in this scale are motor performance, language production, language comprehension, memory, conceptualisation and general knowledge. The scale has been shown to have validity and reliability for use in ID
CAMDEX- DS (adapted from CAMDEX-R) (Ball et al. 2006)	It includes both direct assessments of the person and a structured informant interview. Particular emphasis has been placed on establishing change from the person's best level of functioning

CHAPTER 6

Eating and Drinking Difficulties

Jenny Worsfold[1], Nicky Calow[1] & David Branford[2]

[1]*Leicestershire Partnership NHS Trust, Leicester, UK*
[2]*English Pharmacy Board, Royal Pharmaceutical Society, London, UK*

> Aspiration is only one small factor in dysphagia, and that there are many other signs and symptoms influenced by complex physical, functional, sensory, behavioural and psycho-social factors that impact on assessment and management.
>
> *Lazenby-Paterson et al. (2013)*

Definition

A wide range of factors influence nutrition, hydration, dignity and enjoyment when eating and drinking. 'Eating and drinking difficulties' in this context include dysphagia (swallowing difficulties), loss of independence in self-feeding, difficulties in chewing and swallowing and difficulties in maintaining a safe posture for eating and drinking. This chapter relates to eating and drinking difficulties in adults with intellectual disability (ID) and does not attempt to cover the treatment of children.

The risks of untreated eating and drinking difficulties are malnutrition, dehydration, recurrent chest infections, aspiration pneumonia and death. Other consequences of eating and drinking difficulties include loss of dignity, choice and pleasure.

Clinical presentation

The information in this section is intended as a guide to help the clinician to decide which areas to investigate further in order to make a diagnosis (Table 6.1).

The Frith Prescribing Guidelines for People with Intellectual Disability, Third Edition.
Edited by Sabyasachi Bhaumik, David Branford, Mary Barrett and Satheesh Kumar Gangadharan.
© 2015 John Wiley & Sons, Ltd. Published 2015 by John Wiley & Sons, Ltd.

Table 6.1 Common eating- and drinking-related symptoms and causes to consider.

Symptom domain	Causes to consider
Weight loss	Poor dietary intake
	Poor positioning for eating and drinking
	Infection
	Weight loss as part of another diagnosis, for example, carcinoma
	Gastrointestinal
	• Malabsorption
	• Dietary intolerance
	Poor dentition
	Neuromuscular
	• Loss of motor coordination to feed self
	• Dysphagia/swallowing difficulties
	Iatrogenic
	• Medication side effects
	Mental health factors
	• Depression
	• Psychosis
	• Eating disorder
	• Dementia
	Behavioural issues
	Distraction due to environment
Dehydration	Poor fluid intake (possibly secondary to a dislike of thickened fluids advised for safe swallowing)
	Self-restricting fluid intake to avoid frequent urination or incontinence
	Poor positioning
	Kidney disorders
	Gastrointestinal
	• Malabsorption
	• Poor dentition
	Mental health factors
	• Depression
	• Psychosis
	• Eating disorder
	• Dementia
	Neuromuscular
	• Loss of motor coordination to give self drinks or retain fluid in mouth
Pain on/after eating	Poor dentition
	Oral thrush
	Gastro-oesophageal stricture
	Crico-pharyngeal spasm (feeling of a 'lump in the throat' due to muscle spasm)
	Gastro-oesophageal reflux
	Gastric ulcer/digestive disorders
	Helicobacter pylori infection
	Gallstones

Table 6.1 (*Continued*)

Symptom domain	Causes to consider
Coughing at meals	Poor positioning
	Changes to motor skills or muscle tone
	Overfilling mouth/cramming
	Rushing – either from self or carer
	Failure to chew food properly
	Dysphagia/swallowing disorder
	Gastro-oesophageal reflux
	Crico-pharyngeal spasm
	Pharyngeal pouch
	Medication-induced dysphagia
	Changes to cognition, attention due to a distracting environment, memory or mental health
	Structural changes to anatomy
	Respiratory compromise, for example, COPD, chronic asthma
	Reduced oral sensitivity
Recurrent chest infections	Asthma
	COPD
	Poor oral hygiene
	Dysphagia leading to aspiration of food or drink
	Aspirated reflux
	Aspirated vomit
	Regurgitation
Choking	Respiratory compromise, for example, chronic asthma, COPD
	Inappropriate food texture
	Reduced oral sensitivity
	Overfilling mouth/cramming
	Rushing
	Crico-pharyngeal spasm
	Dysphagia/swallowing problems
	Gastric reflux
Food loss from mouth, food on clothes	Poor positioning
	Loss of motor skills/coordination of motor skills
	Abnormal muscle tone (increased or decreased)
	Tremor, including medication induced
	Reduced oral sensitivity

Conditions associated with eating and drinking difficulties and ID

A number of ID conditions are associated with eating and drinking difficulties. Table 6.2 is adapted with kind permission from Chadwick and Jolliffe (2009; NPSA).

Table 6.2 Conditions associated with eating and drinking difficulties.

Down syndrome, Williams syndrome, Fragile X syndrome, Rubinstein–Taybi syndrome	• Associated oro-pharyngeal structural problems involving the palate, teeth and tongue
Cerebral palsy, epilepsy, Rett syndrome and Noonan syndrome	• Motor processing difficulties giving rise to muscle spasm, changes in muscle tone or muscle coordination, including abnormal tongue movements
General intellectual disability issues	• Higher levels of poor oral health are recorded among people with ID. Respiratory pathogens present in the dental plaque of individuals with very poor dental hygiene may be aspirated and predispose the individual to the development of lung infections • Dependence on others for food and drink • ID and/or history of institutionalisation making the person more susceptible to choking incidents, for example, eating too quickly and cramming food

Table 6.3 Medication-induced dysphagia.

Problem	Example drug groups
Decreased salivation causes dry mouth that can make food bolus 'sticky' and increase risk of choking	Tricyclic antidepressants, some antipsychotics, anticholinergics
Increased salivation causing drooling and has potential to cause choking episodes particularly where swallowing is already compromised	Some antipsychotics, especially clozapine
Tremor	Typical antipsychotics but can also arise with antidepressants
Loss of appetite	SSRI and related antidepressants
Reduced tone of swallowing muscles, difficulty in beginning/coordinating muscle movements that allow passage of food bolus from mouth to stomach	Muscle-relaxants such as benzodiazepines and baclofen

Prevalence

It is difficult to find reliable reports on the prevalence of dysphagia in adults with ID, in part because its definition may include different stages of eating and drinking difficulties.

Studies have reported an estimated prevalence of 5–8% in community samples of adults with ID, up to 30% in hospital samples; in addition, the ID population has been found to have a higher incidence of asphyxiation compared to the general population.

Lung inflammation caused by solids or liquids, and foreign bodies in the windpipe, was involved in 1,048 deaths (14% of those identifiable) of people with learning disabilities or possibly associated conditions. In other people they were involved in just over 2%.

[UK data] Glover and Ayub 2010

The frequency of dysphagia among people with mental health difficulties is reported variously between reported variously between 8 (Chadwick and Jolliffe 2009) and 49% Sheppard and Hochman (1989, cited in Sheppard 2006) (Table 6.3).

Algorithm 6.1 explains best practice in the UK in identifying and treating eating and drinking difficulties in people with ID.

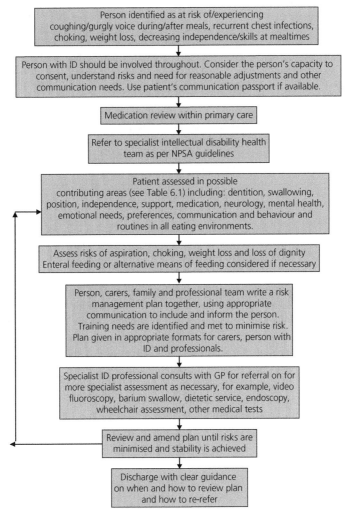

Algorithm 6.1 Algorithm for management of swallowing difficulties in people with intellectual disability.

Illustrative case study 6.1

Meena, a 35-year-old lady with severe ID with challenging behaviour, athetoid cerebral palsy, skeletal changes and visual impairment, visits her general practitioner for an annual health check. Her carers report that she has suffered three chest infections in the last 6 months and over that time, her weight has dropped from 45 kg (BMI = 18 kg/m²) to 40 kg (BMI = 16 kg/m²).

The GP reviews medication and physical health and refers Meena to the dietetic service for nutritional advice and to the specialist ID health team for review of her eating and drinking management.

- The dietitian recommends regular meals and snacks, food fortification and prescription of oral nutritional supplements.

Input from the ID specialist team for Meena is as follows:

- A speech and language therapist (SLT) assesses and finds a risk of aspiration from reduced oral skills and uncoordinated swallow. Using Meena's communication passport, Meena is involved in agreeing food and drinks that are more safely swallowed that she enjoys. A detailed plan of support is written detailing the texture modifications made, verbal support and pacing needed to reduce risks.

    Meena is taking psychotropic medication that can cause dry mouth. The ID psychiatrist changes her medication from haloperidol and procyclidine to risperidone, which gives less severe symptoms of dry mouth.

- A physiotherapist reassesses Meena's stability for eating and drinking and makes adjustments to her chair to improve trunk stability, in turn improving head control.

- An occupational therapist reassesses and recommends a more effective cup to prevent fluid loss but allow thickened fluid through the spout.

Managing nutritional needs

The NICE guideline on nutrition support in adults (http://pathways.nice.org.uk/pathways/nutrition-support-in-adults) recommends that all individuals in nursing and residential homes and in hospital (in- and outpatients) should be screened for the risk of developing malnutrition. This can be done by using the Malnutrition Universal Screening Tool (MUST) (Elia 2003) or another validated tool.

Any person at risk should be monitored closely. This may include weight, food and fluid intake charts and blood biochemistry. Referral to local nutrition and dietetic services should be considered.

Advice about regular meals and snacks and food fortification should normally be used initially, with oral nutritional supplements being prescribed in line with 'Guiding principles for improving the systems and process for oral nutritional supplement use' (National Prescribing Centre 2012; UK) or local medicine management guidance as appropriate. If this fails to arrest weight loss, then consideration should be given to alternative methods of supplementing dietary intake (e.g. nasogastric or gastrostomy tube feeding).

Illustrative case study 6.1 (*Continued*)

> The management plan is updated with a clear support plan for carers. Meena's condition remains stable throughout the summer; however, as winter approaches, her chest infections recur, and she again begins to lose weight. Meena's carers contact the SLT for advice, as per her support plan, as there are risks of aspiration from:
> - Respiratory compromise (scoliosis affecting spine and reducing lung capacity)
> - Pharyngeal dysphagia
> - Inability to maintain a stable position
> - Reflux from compromised positioning
> - Weight loss
>
> The SLT liaises with the GP and refers for video fluoroscopy to assess swallowing in detail. No further management techniques are found to lessen the risks of aspiration from the dysphagia. The team works with the GP to assess the lady's capacity to make a decision about whether to consider enteral feeding and conclude that she does not have capacity to make this choice and therefore this will be a best interest decision. The family is also involved in this decision. The benefits and risks for Meena are considered, and the GP refers to gastroenterology department for assessment. In addition, a community ID nurse becomes involved to support Meena and her family. Meena is referred to the home enteral feeding dietitians for them to explain the risks and benefits of enteral feeding and how this would be used in practice and support the carers.
>
> The gastroenterologist reports that he is willing to place an enteral feeding tube, so another best interest meeting is held where it is agreed to proceed. Meena is taken to meet someone who already has a percutaneous endoscopic gastrostomy (PEG) fitted to understand the experience as far as possible. The dietitian and nurse support patient recovery and training of carers. The SLT identifies safe amounts of preferred food that can continue to be taken orally to minimise risk and maintain quality of life, and the management plan is adjusted accordingly.
>
> A clear care plan is formulated by the whole team involving patient and family and is implemented in all eating environments. The team and GP review the patient until stable. On discharge, all carers are made aware of the process for review and how to re-refer.

Reducing risks

As described in the case study, strategies to reduce the risk of aspiration can be far reaching including changes to position, stability, support, medication, independence and environment. Texture modification can be effective but can also be intrusive and distressing and so should not be considered in isolation and without considering less intrusive means.

Texture modification

Texture modification can reduce the risk of aspiration and may be recommended by an SLT after assessment of the person's oromotor and swallowing ability. Changes to the texture of food can be distressing for a person, so it is essential to include and involve the person as much as possible in understanding their needs

and take into account the person's preferences. The National Patient Safety Agency (2011) (http://www.thenacc.co.uk/assets/downloads/170/Food% 20Descriptors%20for%20Industry%20Final%20-%20USE.pdf) agreed a suite of texture descriptors to which food can be modified from normal texture. These are:
- Fork-mashable diet
- Premashed diet
- Thick puree
- Thin puree

Thickening drinks

Thickeners may be indicated for drinks as a means of reducing risk by creating a cohesive bolus, which moves more slowly and improves bolus control. The SLT will usually contact the prescriber to request this. The dosage is dependent on the desired effect on the fluid. Fluid textures in the UK are governed by the National Descriptors, written in 2002 (Tables 6.4 and 6.5).

Table 6.4 Based on National Descriptors for Texture Modification in Adults. British Dietetic Association and Royal College of Speech and language therapists Joint Working Party (2002).

Description	Normal	Naturally thick	Stage 1	Stage 2	Stage 3
Intended thickness	Water, tea coffee, squash	Milk, some supplements, milkshake, smoothies	Can be drunk through straw or cup. Leaves thin coat on back of spoon	Cannot be drunk through a straw. Can be drunk from cup. Leaves thick coating on back of spoon	Cannot be drunk through straw or cup. Needs to be taken with spoon

Table 6.5 Practicalities of thickener use (based on clinician experience).

Type	Method	Comments	Examples
Starch based	Powder is added to pre-made drink in cup or jug	Thickener may settle on standing, so needs stirring before each mouthful. Appears grainy. Can be difficult to mix with milk products	Fresenius Kabi Thick & Easy™ Nestle RESOURCE® THICKENUP®
Xanthan gum based	Powder added according to instructions	Drink looks unmodified in cup Once made up, retains texture seemingly indefinitely. Good for clear drinks	NUTRICIA Nutilis Clear RESOURCE® THICKENUP CLEAR®
Pre-thickened drinks	None	Portable, ready mixed. Ideal, consistent texture. May have cost implications	Slō Drinks® Nutilis drinks

Three stages of thickness are identified, the naming of which is subjective, and currently subject to much debate. Thickener use can add calories and change salt levels in fluids and must be considered by the prescriber for each person.

Management of saliva

People with ID may have difficulty managing saliva for a number of reasons. Decreased tone and difficulty coordinating facial muscles can result in the accumulation of saliva in the anterior oral cavity, which can then flow out of the mouth. Decreased sensory awareness may also inhibit recognition of pooling of saliva and the person may not be aware of the need to swallow, thus saliva management is impaired (Table 6.6).

Table 6.6 Treatment options for the management of hypersalivation.

Option	By whom?	Limitations and advantages
Sensitisation works to help a person become more aware of saliva pooling and to swallow it	Speech and language therapist	Depends on capacity and insight of person and ability to initiate a swallow Limited success. Can be combined with other treatments. Non-invasive
Improving posture to prevent saliva from falling forwards out of the mouth/ positive positioning to encourage saliva escape and reduce pooling	Physiotherapist	Depends on ability and opportunity to maintain posture Can be combined with other treatments. Non-invasive
Functional approach	Carer	Use bandana bibs, sweat bands or wipes. The person may not remember to wipe or swallow but verbal prompts from a carer may be sufficient
Hyoscine sublingually/ patches	Primary Care Physician	Decreased salivation makes mastication effortful and reduces moistening effect on food, which increases the risk of choking or aspiration of dry food. Food should be moistened with gravies and sauces and table sauces Reducing the amount of saliva produced can increase the concentration of bacteria in the saliva, making it more potent if aspirated and decreasing its cleansing effect. Saliva and secretions can become sticky and are difficult to clear and swallow. The mouth can feel dry and uncomfortable, making swallowing effortful. Risk is increased if the person's cough is weak
Botulinum toxin injections	Surgeon	Intrusive, costly, needs assessment of consent

(Continued)

Table 6.6 (*Continued*)

Option	By whom?	Limitations and advantages
Surgical diversion of salivary glands	Surgeon	Surgical diversion of salivary glands may be considered as a last resort, only after patient has failed to respond effectively to drug treatment and physical therapy The options available are: • Excision of the submandibular gland • Parotid duct diversion • Relocation of the submandibular ducts • Excision of the submandibular glands As the surgery is an intrusive procedure, there may be added risks of anaesthesia and post-operative complications including haemorrhage and pain Capacity assessments may be required prior to proceeding with surgery

Saliva that is not swallowed can also remain in the mouth, causing congestion of breathing, gagging, vomiting, coughing and aspiration. If oral hygiene is compromised or saliva flow reduced by medication, the person's saliva may become concentrated in bacteria and is more likely to cause aspiration pneumonia if aspirated (Langmore 2002).

Choking

People with ID are at a higher risk of choking than the general population (Samuels and Chadwick 2006; Thacker et al. 2007). This is due to several factors including difficulties in chewing, dysphagia, medication effects and behaviours such bolting food and pica (eating non-food items). Those with autism spectrum disorders, mental illness such as paranoia and dementia and those suffering from the effects of institutionalisation can be susceptible to changes to routines and obsessions that can influence the speed of eating and range of food accepted.

Treatment options range from improving eating pace, changes to the eating environment, increased support and medication review while involving the person in their care plan wherever possible. The ID specialist health team can support carers with clinical observation and assessment and behaviour care plans and by providing training for staff or carers in understanding dysphagia management.

Swallowing medication

People with ID may find it difficult to swallow tablets for a number of reasons. Assessment as to the reason for the swallowing difficulty should consider the following causations:
- Anatomical: for example, palatal malformations or gastrostomy feeding due to dysphagia.
- Physiological: dry mouth, feeling that tablet is stuck in the throat and reflux symptoms.
- Other: concern over size of tablet, dislike for tablets, change in tablet appearance and 'always' had liquid preparations. People with autism spectrum disorders may be particularly restrictive in their willingness to embrace changes in new medications (e.g. may only accept 'blue ones').

Management strategies

- Identify if the tablet can be crushed/dissolved in water (always check with pharmacy before tablet is crushed/cut).
- Check if there is a route for administration through PEG, if PEG is inserted.
- Choose alternatives such as orodispersible tablets, liquid and other preparations such as chronospheres.
- If the above fails, consider a capacity assessment and best interest decision for administering medication covertly. Document clearly the members of the multi-disciplinary team (MDT), the capacity assessment, the reason for the best interest decision and when to review and involve the family/carers in this decision.

Feeding tubes

Individuals with severe swallowing difficulties may require complete avoidance of oral food, fluids and medications and therefore may have either a nasogastric tube or insertion of a gastrostomy tube. There are two types of gastrostomy:
1 PEG tube; this is a tube inserted directly into the stomach. This is the more common type of gastrostomy.
2 Percutaneous endoscopic gastrostomy with a jejunal extension (PEGJ) (because PEJ are rarely used, we think PEGJ is better mentioned instead). PEGJ is used where people are prone to reflux and sickness or at high risk of aspiration.

The use of enteral feeding tubes has increased both for short- and long-term feedings due to increasing awareness of the importance of ensuring adequate nutritional and fluid intake for promotion and maintenance of good health. Gastrostomy tubes provide a means of improving nutritional intake when oral intake is very poor or when there is restricted access to the GI tract either due to swallowing difficulties or an obstruction. Dietitians are essential members of the MDT who ensure people with gastrostomy tubes receive adequate fluid and nutrition and will prescribe a diet based on individual requirements and relevant disease states. The gastrostomy tube itself needs to be looked after to maintain good hygiene and prevent infection, as well as to reduce the risk of the tube blocking or coming out.

Consider the feeding regime when prescribing medication. Ideally, there should be a gap around medication administration (e.g. medications such as phenytoin require 2 hours either side of administration as they will bind to proteins in feeds). Some medication will react with feeds to cause insoluble precipitates that could potentially block the tube.

The following points should be considered when prescribing medication:

- Osmotic diarrhoea from liquid medicines that contain sorbitol. The dose is cumulative so the risk increases with the more medicines there are. The patient can experience painful cramping with the diarrhoea.
- Poor absorption, especially when feeding into the jejunum, as the medication may enter the GI tract too low down to be adequately absorbed.
- Altered bioavailability when converting from some tablets to liquids.
- Changing from a modified-release preparation to a liquid will mean reduced doses but more frequent intervals.
- Risk of tube blocking from viscous liquids.
- Risk of the medication binding to the plastic tube – these medications will require dilution prior to administration.

A person with ID on a modified or enteral diet will often require careful thought around choice of formulation. It might be that there is an alternative route of administration available, for example, changing tablets to patches. Many liquid formulations are relatively thick and will be safe for administration to an individual requiring a modified diet; however, it may be necessary to thicken liquid medication. If there is no liquid formulation available, tablets may need to be crushed or capsules opened and then mixed with water for administration. Altering the manufacturer's formulation of a medication by thickening, crushing or opening capsules can alter the process by which it is absorbed into the body. Modified release medications must never be crushed or chewed (Wright et al. 2012) (Table 6.7).

For people with ID with enteral tubes who receive all fluid, nutrition and medications via the gastrostomy, it is important to ensure that the feeding regimen does not adversely affect the medication, for example, phenytoin can

Table 6.7 Some medications that should never be crushed or opened.

Formulations with any kind of enteric coating – these medications could be an irritant or be affected by environmental conditions

Modified- or sustained-release formulations – the pharmacokinetics of these formulations will be altered

Hormones or cytotoxic medications – due to the risk of harm to the person administering the medication

Nitrates – due to the theoretical risk of explosion

bind to proteins in feeds. It is important that carers of individuals with swallowing difficulties/gastrostomy tubes have clear guidance on how to safely administer medication, this will require multidisciplinary input from speech and language therapy, dietetics and pharmacy as well as the relevant prescribers, and it might be useful to provide written information. Many pharmaceutical companies will have information on administering their medication to individuals with swallowing difficulties/gastrostomy tubes, but will emphasise that they will not have stability information and that it is an unlicensed use. There are a number of useful reference sources that have information on prescribing and administration of medications for people with swallowing difficulties/gastrostomy tubes as well as very useful monographs for individual medication including antiepileptic and psychotropic medications.

Guidance on the administration of medication via PEG tubes

There are many guidelines and resources available to guide the administration of particular medication. For that reason, we have not provided a table of such guidance in this edition of the Frith Guidelines. Regularly updated sources are available and include:
- UKMi. (2009, December; partial revision January 2010). Medicines Q&A 294.1a: Therapeutic options for patients unable to take solid oral dosage forms. Available online at: https://view.officeapps.live.com/op/view.aspx?src=http%3A%2F%2Fwww.medicinesresources.nhs.uk%2Fupload%2Fdocuments%2FEvidence%2FMedicines%2520Q%2520%26%2520A%2FNW_QA294_3_Solidoraldosageformsalternatives.doc
- White, R., Bradnam, V. (2007) Handbook of medication administration via enteral feeding tubes. London: RPS Publishing.
- Smyth, J. (2006). The NEWT guidelines for administration of medication to patients with enteral feeding tubes or swallowing difficulties. Wrexham: North East Wales NHS Trust.
- Australian don't rush to crush handbook: Therapeutic options for people unable to swallow solid oral medicines. http://www.shpa.org.au/lib/pdf/publications/DRTC (accessed 7 January 2015).

If medication is to be administered via a PEG tube, the following is recommended:
- Make the prescriber aware that:
  - The person has a PEG tube.
  - The formulations of the medications prescribed are appropriate to go into the PEG tube.
- Not all liquids are suitable for administration via a PEG tube because they may be too thick.

- Medications that must not be crushed/opened to be administered via a PEG tube include:
  - Enteric-coated tablets – these tablets have a coating on them to either protect the medication or to prevent gastric irritation.
  - Controlled-/modified-/sustained-release, long-acting, retard formulations or chrono-formulations – these formulations allow decreased dosing frequency and encourage more consistent blood levels of a medication.
  - Hormones and cytotoxics – because of possible harm to the person administering the medication.

The following points should be remembered when administering medications via a PEG tube:

- They should not be added to a feed.
- Only one should be administered at a time. They should not be mixed.
- A 50 mL syringe should be used to reduce the likelihood of strong pressure rupturing the tube.
- Cooled boiled water should be used when dispersing tablets and flushing the tube:
  - Flush tube with a minimum of 15 mL of water between medications.
  - Flush tube with 50 mL of water after administration of the last medication.
  - Always flush the PEG tube pre/post and between medicines. The exact volume of water required for the flushes will be calculated on an individual basis by the dietitian, depending on tolerance.

It is often easier to prepare all of the medications for administration in an area away from the person with ID so that they can then be administered consecutively with the minimum amount of disruption.

Directions for administration of tablets via a feeding tube

Crushing tablets
1 Crush the tablets in a tablet crusher.
2 Add 15–30 mL of cooled boiled water to the crusher and mix with the powder.
3 Draw up the solution in an oral or bladder syringe or suitable administration container.
4 Rinse out the crusher with cooled boiled water using the same syringe and dispense into the suitable administration container.

Dispersible/disintegrating tablets
Tablets may disintegrate in water without crushing. If this is the case, the tablet should be prepared as follows:
1 Place intact tablet into the barrel of an oral/bladder syringe.
2 Replace the plunger and draw up 10–15 mL of cooled boiled water.
3 Replace the cap and allow tablet to dissolve.

4 Shake well and administer dose down the enteral feeding tube.
5 Flush the tube post-dose with 15–30 mL of water.

Effervescent tablets

Tablets will effervesce and disperse when placed in water. The resulting gases need to be allowed to escape.

1 Pour 50 mL cooled boiled water into a glass/beaker.
2 Add the tablet to the water.
3 Wait for the effervescent reaction to finish.
4 Swirl the solution and draw it all up into a 50 mL oral/bladder syringe.
5 Administer the dose down the enteral feeding tube.

What not to do with tablets:

Do not:

- Crush the tablet in a plastic container other than the tablet crusher supplied as the medication may adhere to the plastic.
- Use boiling water to dissolve tablets as it may affect bioavailability.
- Leave oral medications unattended in syringes.
- Administer any medication that you have not prepared yourself.

Discussion case study 6.2

Adam is a 40-year-old man with moderate ID and Down syndrome. He attends his annual health check at the GP surgery. The health check identifies he is losing weight.

On questioning, it becomes clear that Adam is struggling to eat a full meal and coughs on occasion when eating.

- What is the role of the GP in this case?
- Who might the GP refer to?
- What recommendations would you expect to be made by:
  a) A dietitian
  b) The ID health team

References

British Dietetic Association and Royal College of Speech and Language Therapists (2002). http://www.thenacc.co.uk/assets/downloads/170/Food%20Descriptors%20for%20Industry%20Final%20-%20USE.pdf (accessed 20 May 2015).

Chadwick, D. D., Jolliffe, J. (2009) A descriptive investigation of dysphagia in adults with intellectual disabilities. *Journal of Intellectual Disability Research*, 53:29–43.

Elia, M. (2003) Nutritional screening for adults: a multidisciplinary responsibility. Development and use of the 'Malnutrition Universal Screening Tool' (MUST) for adults. The 'MUST' report. British Association for Parenteral and Enteral Nutrition (BAPEN), Redditch.

Glover, G., Ayub, M. (2010, June) How people with learning disabilities die. Improving health and lives observatory report DoH. http://www.improvinghealthandlives.org.uk/uploads/doc/vid_9033_IHAL2010-06%20Mortality.pdf (accessed 7 January 2015).

Langmore, S.E., Skarupski, K.A., Park, P.S., Fries, B.E. (2002) Predictors of Aspiration Pneumonia in Nursing Home Residents. *Dysphagia*, 17(4):298–307.

Lazenby-Paterson, T., Brown, L., Crawford, H. (2013, September) Striking the right balance in ALD. *Royal College of Speech and Language Therapists Bulletin*, 10–11.

National Institute for Health and Care Excellence (NICE) (2006) Nutrition support in adult. http://pathways.nice.org.uk/pathways/nutrition-support-in-adults (accessed 20 May 2015).

National Prescribing Centre (2012) Quality standard for nutrition support in adults. http://www.nice.org.uk/guidance/qs24/resources/guidance-quality-standard-for-nutrition-support-in-adults-pdf (accessed 3 March 2015).

NPSA (2011) National descriptors for texture modification in adults. BDA/RCSLT, Birmingham.

Samuels, R., Chadwick, D. D. (2006) Predictors of asphyxiation risk in adults with intellectual disabilities and dysphagia. *Journal of Intellectual Disability Research* 50(5):362–370.

Sheppard, J. J. (2006) Developmental disability and swallowing disorders in adults. In *Dysphagia: Foundations: Theory and Practice* (eds J. Cichero and B. Murdoch), pp. 299–318. Wiley & Sons Ltd., Chichester.

Sheppard, J. J., Hochman, R. (1989) Clinical symptoms of dysphagia in mentally retarded individuals. Paper presented at the American Speech-Language-Hearing Association Annual Convention, St. Louis, November.

Thacker, A., Abdelnoor, A., Anderson, C., White, S., Hollins, S. (2007) Indicators of choking risk in adults with learning disabilities: A questionnaire survey and interview study. *Disability and Rehabilitation*, 30(15):1131–1138.

Wright, D., Beavon, N., Branford, D., et al. (2012) Guideline for the identification and management of swallowing difficulties in adults with learning disability *RCGP*. http://www.guidelines.co.uk/gastrointestinal_wp_dysphagia_2012#.VXfjaPmqpBc (accessed 20 May 2015).

Further reading

Boaden, E., Davies, S., Storey, L., Watkins, C. (2006) Inter-professional dysphagia framework. Royal College of Speech and Language Therapists, University of Lancashire, Lancashire. http://www.rcslt.org/members/publications/publications2/Framework_pdf (accessed 20 May 2015).

Dignity in Care (2010) Dignity Champions action pack – nutrition and assistance with eating. http://www.dignityincare.org.uk/_library/Dignity_Champions_Action_Pack_-_Nutrition_and_Assistance_with_eating.pdf (accessed 21 June 2013).

Hampshire Safeguarding Adults Board (2012) Reducing the risk of choking for people with a learning disability. A multi-agency review in Hampshire. http://documents.hants.gov.uk/adultservices/safeguarding/Reducingtheriskofchokingforpeoplewithalearningdisability.pdf (accessed 7 January 2015).

Helen, C. (2007) *Eating well: Children and adults with learning disabilities.* Caroline Walker Trust, Abbots Langley.

Heslop, P., Blair, P., Fleming, P., Hoghton, M., Marriott, A., Russ, L. (2013) *Confidential inquiry into premature deaths of people with learning disabilities (CIPOLD).* Bristol University, Bristol.

Langmore, S., Terpenning, M. S., Schork, A., et al. (1998) Predictors of aspiration pneumonia: How important is dysphagia? *Dysphagia* 13:69–81.

Mencap (2007) Death by indifference. Mencap, London.

Mencap (2012) 74 deaths and counting. Mencap, London.

Michael, J. (2008) Healthcare for all. The report of the Michael enquiry. Department of Health, London. http://webarchive.nationalarchives.gov.uk/20130107105354/http:/www.dh.gov.

uk/en/Publicationsandstatistics/Publications/PublicationsPolicyAndGuidance/DH_099255 (accessed 3 March 2015).

National Institute for Health and Clinical Excellence (2004) Dyspepsia: Management of dyspepsia in adults in primary care. NICE clinical guidance 17. http://www.nice.org.uk/guidance/cg17 (accessed 7 January 2015).

National Institute for Health and Clinical Excellence (2012) Quality standard for nutrition support in adults. NICE quality standard 24. http://guidance.nice.org.uk/QS24 (accessed 7 January 2015).

National Patient Safety Agency (2007) Problems swallowing? http://www.thenacc.co.uk/assets/downloads/170/Food%20Descriptors%20for%20Industry%20Final%20-%20USE.pdf (accessed 3 March 2015).

NPSA, RCSLT, BDA, NNNG and Hospital Caterers Association (2011, April) Dysphagia diet food texture descriptors. http://www.thenacc.co.uk/assets/downloads/170/Food%20Descriptors%20for%20Industry%20Final%20-%20USE.pdf (accessed 3 March 2015).

Watson, F., Chadwick, D., Stobbart, V., Kelly, A. (2006) Dysphagia in adults with learning disabilities: findings from the dysphagia working party NPSA.

CHAPTER 7

Sleep Disorders

David Bramble[1] & Reza Kiani[2]

[1]*Shropshire Community Health NHS Trust, Shrewsbury, UK*
[2]*Leicestershire Partnership NHS Trust, Leicester, UK*

> True silence is the rest of the mind, and is to the spirit what sleep is to the body, nourishment and refreshment.
>
> *William Penn*

People with intellectual disabilities (ID) often present with persistent sleep difficulties which can, in themselves, contribute significantly to their overall handicap, but these mostly represent the result of poor sleep habits and can respond well to healthy sleep-promoting advice and behavioural strategies (see below). However, within this population there are also over-representations of underlying physical conditions that can significantly disrupt sleep such as abnormal brain development, brain damage, epilepsy and also disturbance of the function of the neurological pathways involving melatonin and other neurotransmitters that modulate the sleep–wake cycle. A variety of other medical and psychiatric factors may also produce marked sleep disruption. All of these factors will be examined in this chapter.

Definition

The cardinal clinical symptoms and signs of sleep disorders fall into five principal categories, which commonly overlap:
1 Difficulty falling sleep (initial insomnia)
2 Difficulty staying asleep (broken sleep)
3 Waking too early in the morning (late insomnia)
4 Daytime sleepiness
5 Unusual behaviours seen only in and around the sleep period (parasomnias)

The Frith Prescribing Guidelines for People with Intellectual Disability, Third Edition.
Edited by Sabyasachi Bhaumik, David Branford, Mary Barrett and Satheesh Kumar Gangadharan.
© 2015 John Wiley & Sons, Ltd. Published 2015 by John Wiley & Sons, Ltd.

The International Classification of Sleep Disorders, Second Edition (ICSD-2, 2005) has classified sleep disorders into eight categories:

1 Insomnias
2 Sleep-related breathing disorders
3 Hypersomnias of central origin not due to a circadian rhythm disorder, sleep-related breathing disorder or other cause of disturbed sleep
4 Circadian rhythm sleep disorders
5 Parasomnias
6 Sleep-related movement disorders
7 Isolated symptoms, apparently normal variants and unresolved issues
8 Other sleep disorders

This chapter concentrates on insomnia and its management but does briefly cover other types of sleep disorder.

Insomnia

The term insomnia is defined as 'a disabling insufficiency of sleep quantity or quality'. When insomnia impairs a person's quality of life, it should be treated. Identification and treatment of any underlying problems resolve the accompanying insomnia in most cases (Table 7.1).

Clinical presentation

Sleep disorders not only represent a significant risk factor for psychiatric illness in the ID population but may also be a major cause of stress among parents and carers, being associated with poor concentration, impaired learning and

Table 7.1 Underlying causes of insomnia.

Poor sleep hygiene	Stressful situations
• Uncomfortable bed	• Grief reactions
• Noisy household	• Change of placement/change of bedroom
• Poor light and temperature adjustment	
• Late evening caffeine	
Physiological conditions	**Psychiatric conditions**
• Old age	• Anxiety disorders
• Pregnancy	• Affective disorders
	• Psychotic disorders
	• Delirium and dementia
Medical and iatrogenic causes	**Medical and iatrogenic causes**
• Pruritis	• Respiratory disorders (dyspnoea)
• Pain	• Nocturia
• Epilepsy	• Thyroid disorders
• Cardiac diseases (heart failure and orthopnoea)	• Alcohol and substance misuse
	• Medications

communication skills and behaviour problems (e.g. self-injurious behaviour, aggression, screaming).

Chronically disturbed sleep can add considerably to the burden of care and is a leading factor in family crises, which may require the involvement of statutory agencies.

Various genetic conditions associated with ID are particularly associated with specific sleep disorders; for example, a high number of people with Down syndrome may have obstructive sleep apnoea because of obesity, short neck, hypotonicity and structural abnormalities of the upper respiratory tract (narrow airways, large adenoid and tonsils, large tongue and small jaw). Obstructive sleep apnoea may occur in other genetic syndromes like Rubinstein–Taybi, Prader–Willi, Angelman and fragile X.

High rates of seizures in this population and use of antiepileptic medications can also produce sleep disruption, which in turn can adversely affect epilepsy control.

Prevalence

Sleep disturbance is common sequelae of a number of developmental conditions. Research shows that nearly all parents of children with Williams syndrome report that their child had sleep difficulties that could have a negative impact on daytime behaviour. Likewise, children with Down syndrome were found to have significantly more difficulty with sleep, with large number of parents reporting that their child seemed tired during the day, indicating inadequate sleep.

When studied during a 4-week period, the overall prevalence of sleep problems in the ID population was found to be approximately 9%, and significant sleep problems were more likely to be associated with mental ill health, problem behaviours, visual impairment and respiratory disease. The prevalence of sleep problems in people with ID has however been reported in various studies as being as high as 15–50%.

Management

The degree of ID and communication difficulties may prevent the person from either realising that there is a problem in the first place or, even if this is recognised, to consider bringing it to the attention of others. A sleep history (Table 7.2), used in combination with a sleep diary, obtained from the carer, provides sufficient information to characterise the person's sleep problem and guides further therapeutic options.

The over-representation of both psychiatric and medical disorders in the ID population requires that all people displaying significant sleep disturbance are also screened for these factors, as they may be either contributing significantly or even causing the presenting problem.

It should be borne in mind that non-pharmacological management of sleep difficulties always takes precedence over the use of medication; however, if these prove insufficient, then consideration of medication alongside non-medication strategies may be appropriate.

Prerequisites for a good night's sleep are a comfortable sleeping environment and a conducive sleep habit. As a growing number of adults with ID are living in more independent settings, with only limited supervision, it is possible that such conditions may be more difficult to achieve. Therefore, it is beholden upon such professionals to be aware of the importance of encouraging healthy sleep habits. There is a large research and clinical literature attesting to the efficacy and tolerability of sleep hygiene (Table 7.3) and behavioural strategies (Table 7.4) in the management of insomnia.

Table 7.2 Sleep history.

- Information on sleep hygiene, bedroom and bedtime routine
- Onset, duration and nature of the problem (e.g. difficulty dropping off, frequent awakening, early morning insomnia, motor activities and snoring during sleep; evidence of daytime hyper-somnolence)
- Effect of insomnia on person, family and/or carer
- Past sleep difficulties and previous treatments
- Psychiatric and medical diagnosis
- Current medication regime
- Family history of sleep problems
- Medication and alcohol misuse

Table 7.3 Sleep hygiene.

- Encourage daily exercise
- Avoid daytime napping
- Reduce caffeine and alcohol intake before bedtime
- Eliminate factors that impede sleep (watching TV and games consoles and use of computers in bedroom)
- Use the bed just for sleeping
- Set and maintain a regular routine of rising and retiring at the same time every day (bedtime routine)
- Ensure sleeping environment is conducive to sleep (comfortable bed, quiet, dark and at the right temperature)

Table 7.4 Behavioural strategies.

- Removal of carer's over-attention to the person at bedtime
- Behavioural extinction and stimulus control (increasing the association between bed and sleep by eliminating sleep-incompatible activities from the bedroom)
- Chronotherapy for sleep phase disorders (progressive incremental adjustment of bedtime to the desired time)

Illustrative case study 7.1

> A 24-year-old lady with severe ID as a result of a developmental brain abnormality (holoprosencephaly) and treatment-resistant epilepsy was referred by her general practitioner for management of severe self-injury and aggression.
>
> During history taking, parents informed the psychiatrist that she was also suffering from severe sleep problems, in the form of staying awake at night-time but having frequent naps during daytime. On further probing, it became obvious that all these started when her college course finished a year ago.
>
> Further assessment confirmed an accompanying autism spectrum disorder, and as she was already on several medications for the management of treatment-resistant epilepsy, it was decided that a community nurse should be involved to work around sleep hygiene and behavioural strategies in the management of her sleep difficulties.
>
> A referral was also made to social services who then commissioned daily structured community-based activities, providing both mental stimulation and physical exercise. A review in 6 months' time showed a dramatic improvement in sleep pattern and challenging behaviour without any need for pharmacological management.

Medication strategies

Although not evidence-based practice, clinicians still use low doses of various antipsychotic (e.g. chlorpromazine), antidepressant (e.g. trazodone) or antihistamine (e.g. promethazine) medications for night-time sedation in people with psychiatric illness and/or ID. However, in recent years, owing to greater recognition of the importance of treating sleep difficulties effectively by the wider application of non-pharmacological techniques, medications now have only limited and specific roles in the management of the commonest sleep disorders and are usually reserved for use in crises and in refractory cases.

Melatonin

This naturally occurring substance has been successfully used in the management of sleep–wake cycle disturbances in people with ID, visual impairment and autism spectrum disorders.

There is no compelling evidence that controlled-release or other long-acting formulations yield any additional benefits, particularly when used to address repeated night-waking problems. A meta-analysis in 2006 concluded that melatonin was not effective in treating secondary sleep disorders or sleep disorders accompanying sleep restriction such as jet lag and shift work disorder, but at the same time found its short-term use safe.

A clinical review of studies available on the efficacy of melatonin has revealed that melatonin is most useful at reducing sleep latency; however, it is not consistently effective in reducing habitual night-waking patterns. However, a randomised placebo-controlled study in people with ID found that melatonin improved overall sleep by decreasing sleep latency, advancing sleep onset and increasing total time of sleep.

Another study on three people with moderate to severe ID did not reveal any significant effects on quantity and quality of sleep following administration of melatonin, but showed a change in circadian rhythm along with improvement of behaviour problems. A recent randomised double-masked placebo-controlled trial in children with neurodevelopmental disorders showed that melatonin reduced sleep onset latency but at the same time was associated with earlier waking time than placebo. It also showed improved outcomes in child behaviour and family functioning. Adverse effects were also reported as mild and similar to what were reported in the placebo group. Melatonin is not generally considered to produce tolerance, rebound insomnia or dependency, problems often associated with other sedative hypnotics. A dose as low as 0.5 mg can be effective in some cases.

The only melatonin product currently licensed in the UK is Circadin, a modified release preparation licensed for the treatment of primary insomnia in people over the age of 55. Although melatonin is commonly used in practice in children and adolescent mental health services and in ID settings, regular review and accurate documentation of its beneficial as well as its side effects are strongly recommended.

Illustrative case study 7.2

Michelle is an 18-year-old girl with a diagnosis of moderate ID and ADHD who has recently been transferred from child and adolescent mental health services to the adult ID service. In addition to stimulant treatment for the management of her ADHD, Michelle takes liquid melatonin 6 mg nocte, which was previously found effective for initial insomnia.

On review, it was unclear whether Michelle was still benefitting from melatonin treatment. She and her parents agreed to taper the medication to see if it was still required. Her parents were reminded of non-pharmacological strategies and advised to continue adhering to these while gradually tapering her medication. Her other medications were kept unchanged.

When seen again in 3 months' time, there were reports of a return of difficulties in getting off to sleep and an increase in her challenging behaviour during the day. A report from college also showed deterioration in her concentration, alongside tiredness and irritability. There were no other accompanying factors explaining the relapse of insomnia and challenging behaviour, except the recent reduction in dose of melatonin.

It was therefore agreed with her and her parents to put up the dose of melatonin back to the previous regime to see if this produced any improvement in her sleep pattern and challenging behaviour. A telephone review after 2 weeks reported positive feedback on the effectiveness of this strategy, and therefore, melatonin was continued and a further review was scheduled within 6 months.

Sedative hypnotics

Older sedatives including barbiturates, antihistamines and chloral hydrate have been largely superseded by shorter-acting benzodiazepines and the so-called z-medications: zopiclone, zolpidem and zaleplon. These medications are licensed to be used in insomnia.

Use of short-term, prn benzodiazepines and 'z-medications' should be a last resort in the management of insomnia, as they may cause paradoxical excitement, daytime sleepiness, tolerance and dependence and their withdrawal may be accompanied by rebound insomnia, anxiety symptoms, low mood, suicidal ideation and seizures. If hypnotics are to be used regularly, they are preferably to be prescribed for 1 week and no longer than 2–4 weeks (Table 7.5).

A minority of patients, often co-morbid for autism or visual impairment, may require long-term drug treatment, in these circumstances their ongoing need for such treatment should be reviewed at least annually. In rare circumstances, people whose quality of life has been impaired by a long-standing disturbed sleep pattern might benefit from long-term use of hypnotic agents. If hypnotic agents are to be used, it is better to use long-acting agents (e.g. nitrazepam and zopiclone) for frequent night-time or early morning wakening. Short-acting agents (e.g. temazepam, zolpidem and zaleplon) are best for the management of initial insomnia; however, their use should be frequently reviewed and documented in the notes.

Older people, frail individuals and people with signs and symptoms of hepatic impairment are particularly sensitive to the adverse effects of hypnotic agents. Because they might experience ataxia, confusional state and falls, cautious use of lower doses of short-acting hypnotics are preferred in these populations. Hypnotics should not be used in children.

Table 7.5 Summary of NICE guidance for hypnotic use.

- Use non-pharmacological approaches first
- Use the cheapest medication first
- There are no differences in the efficacy of z-medications, and if one is not effective, the others should not be used
- Switch from one z-medication to another if there is an adverse effect directly related to that particular medication
- Use the minimum effective dose
- Use prn (as needed) medication every second or third night if required, rather than regularly
- Do not continue longer than 4 weeks
- Discuss the discontinuation with the person and taper and stop it gradually
- Warn the person of withdrawal symptoms and rebound insomnia
- Advise on the interaction with alcohol and other sedative agents
- Do not use in hepatic failure, chronic respiratory diseases and people who have a history of substance misuse

Other hypnotics

In the UK, several antihistamines like promethazine have been used for insomnia either by prescription or over the counter. None of the antihistamines have been demonstrated to provide lasting benefits, and they can produce a range of side effects that include morning 'hangover' sleepiness through their long half-life. Therefore, they are not recommended for treating insomnia.

Chloral hydrate, clomethiazole and triclofos sodium are all licensed in the UK for the management of insomnia in the general population, but there are no studies available for their use in the ID population and their use is generally not recommended.

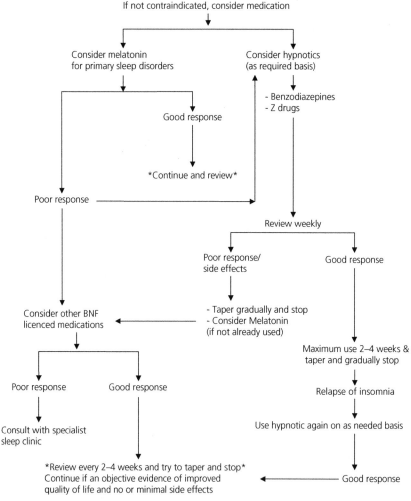

Algorithm 7.1 Insomnia not responding to management of underlying condition and non-pharmacological approaches.

Algorithm 7.1 may be used to decide which sedative hypnotic drug should be used in a patient with refractory insomnia.

Antidepressants

Antidepressants are the medication of choice if sleep difficulties are secondary to depression. They are also effective in the management of daytime sleepiness in narcolepsy and nocturnal enuresis in children, although they have been largely superseded by synthetic desmopressin for the latter indication.

Antipsychotics

All antipsychotics can produce sedation. A person who is already taking this type of medication and has tried other non-medication measures but failed to achieve a normal sleep pattern, the daily dose of antipsychotic can be adjusted so that a higher dose is given in the evenings. It should, however, be noted that the antipsychotics are *not* licensed for the treatment of any specific sleep disorder.

Other sleep disorders

Obstructive sleep apnoea
Obstructive sleep apnoea occurs relatively frequently in people with ID and is commonly associated with the higher rates of clinical obesity encountered in this population. Third-party reports of extremely loud and frequent snoring interspersed by periods of apnoea for a few seconds and daytime sleepiness characterise this condition. The definitive diagnostic tool is polysomnography in a sleep clinic; however, the availability and practicality of using this technique with many people with ID may limit its use. It would be ideal to refer the person to a respiratory physician for further investigation and advice. Reduction in weight, continuous positive airway pressure and surgical correction of structural abnormalities are the principal methods used in the management of this condition. Sedative hypnotics, especially benzodiazepines, are contraindicated owing to the risk of respiratory arrest through smooth muscle relaxation leading to airway collapse.

Hypersomnia
Hypersomnia is defined as excessive daytime sleepiness with impairment of cognitive, social and occupational functioning. Important differential diagnoses are narcolepsy, obstructive sleep apnoea, epilepsy, psychiatric disorders (e.g. seasonal affective disorder (SAD)), alcohol (and other substances) misuse and organic (e.g. endocrine changes and organ failure) and iatrogenic causes (e.g. sedative medications).

As for the management of insomnia, treatment strategies first should concentrate on sleep hygiene and treatment of the underlying cause.

Modafinil (a non-selective noradrenaline and dopamine reuptake inhibitor) has been effectively used in the management of daytime sleepiness in narcolepsy.

Sleep–wake cycle disturbances

The misalignment of the internal sleep–wake circadian clock with environmental day/night patterns and other environmental cues may also result in sleep disorders. This is more common in autism spectrum disorders and in visual impairment. With this kind of sleep disorder, the length of the principal sleep period remains normal but occurs at an undesirable time, either too early (advanced sleep phase disorder) or too late (delayed).

Treating any underlying problem and adhering to rigid sleep hygiene should bring the cycle back to normal. Chronotherapy and light therapy are also useful treatment strategies in the management of sleep phase disorders. A trial of melatonin can be used if non-pharmacological approaches fail to reverse the cycle back to normal.

Parasomnias

Parasomnias (e.g. sleepwalking and sleep terrors) should be differentiated from night-time epilepsy. Where nocturnal epilepsy is suspected, a 24-hour EEG recording is indicated. The main management strategy is to keep the bedroom safe to prevent any physical injuries. Treatment of any accompanying physical or psychiatric illness, family therapy and relaxation techniques may all be helpful. Judicious and short-term use of medication (e.g. clonazepam) can be helpful in suppressing rapid eye movement (REM) sleep and thus any associated parasomnia.

Discussion case study 7.3

> Here is a clinical case scenario the reader may find helpful in applying the knowledge provided in this chapter. A 35-year-old man with mild ID is urgently referred by his GP with a chief complaint of feeling suicidal and only managing to have 2–3 hours of sleep at night. The sleep difficulties have been going on for the last 6 months and began following relationship difficulties with the man's long-term partner, resulting in him having to leave home and move back in with his mother. He has begun feeling very low and threatened several times to take an overdose.
>
> The GP prescribed him prn diazepam 3 months ago, which he began using regularly to help him get off to sleep. On questioning, he also admits to intermittently using cannabis and alcohol to help him settle at night. Despite this, he is still suffering from insomnia and is now saying that he cannot go on like this any longer.
> - What type of sleep disorder is he suffering from?
> - What are the most likely aetiological factors for his insomnia?
> - How would you manage the situation? What are your priorities?

Further reading

American Academy of Sleep Medicine (2005) *International classification of sleep disorders: diagnostic & coding manual*, 2nd edn. American Academy of Sleep Medicine, Westchester, IL.

Annaz D, Hill CM, Ashworth A, et al. (2011) Characterisation of sleep problems in children with Williams syndrome. *Res Dev Disabil*. 32: 164–9.

Barnhill J (2006) The assessment and differential diagnosis of insomnia in people with developmental disability. *Mental Health Aspect Dev Disabil*. 9: 109–18.

Boyle A, Melville CA, Morrison J, et al. (2010) A cohort study of the prevalence of sleep problems in adults with intellectual disabilities. *J Sleep Res*. 19: 42–53.

Braam W, Didden R, Smits M, et al. (2008) Melatonin treatment in individuals with intellectual disability and chronic insomnia: a randomised placebo-controlled study. *J Intellect Disabil Res*. 52(3): 256–64.

Braam W, Smits MG, Didden R, et al. (2009) Exogenous melatonin for sleep problems in individuals with intellectual disability: a meta-analysis. *Dev Med Child Neurol*. 51(5): 340–9.

Bramble D, Freehan C (2005) Psychiatrists' use of melatonin with children. *Child Adolesc Mental Health*. 10(3): 145–9.

British Medical Association and the Royal Pharmaceutical Society of Great Britain. (2013) *British National Formulary. Section 4 – Central nervous system: Hypnotics and anxiolytics*. pp. 218–227. BMJ Publishing Group Ltd. & Pharmaceutical Press, London.

Buscemi N, Vandermeer B, Hooton N, et al. (2006) Efficacy and safety of exogenous melatonin for secondary sleep disorders and sleep disorders accompanying sleep restriction: meta-analysis. *BMJ*. 332: 385.

Carter M, McCaughey E, Annaz D, et al. (2009) Sleep problems in a Down syndrome population. *Arch Dis Child*. 94: 308–10.

Dodd A, Hare DJ, Arshad P (2008) The use of melatonin to treat sleep disorder in adults with intellectual disabilities in community settings – the evaluation of three cases using actigraphy. *J Intellect Disabil Res*. 52: 547–53.

Espie CA (2000) Sleep and disorders of sleep in people with mental retardation. *Curr Opin Psychiatry*. 13(5): 507–11.

Gringras P, Gamble C, Jones AP, et al. (2012) Melatonin for sleep problems in children with neurodevelopmental disorders: randomised double masked placebo controlled trial. *BMJ*. 345: e6664.

Hylkema T, Vlaskamp C (2009) Significant improvement in sleep in people with intellectual disabilities living in residential settings by non-pharmaceutical interventions. *J Intellect Disabil Res* 53(8):695–703.

Jan MMS (2000) Melatonin for the treatment of handicapped children with severe sleep disorders. *Pediatr Neurol*. 23(3): 229–32.

Levanon A, Taksiuk A, Tal A (1999) Sleep characteristics in children with Down syndrome. *J Pediatr*. 134(6): 755–60.

Mendez M, Radtke R (2001) Interaction between sleep and epilepsy. *J Clin Neurophysiol*. 18(2): 106–27.

National Institute for Health and Care Excellence (2004) Guidance on the use of zaleplon, zolpidem and zopiclone for the short-term management of insomnia. NICE Technology appraisal guidance [TA77]. NICE, London. Available at: www.nice.org.uk (accessed 7 January 2015).

Reite M, Ruddy J, Nagel K (2002) *The evaluation and management of sleep disorders*, 3rd edn. American Psychiatric Publishing, Arlington, VA.

Rzepecka H, McKenzie K, McClure I, et al. (2011) Sleep, anxiety and challenging behaviour in children with intellectual disability and/or autism spectrum disorder. *Res Dev Disabil*. 32(6): 2758–66.

Sajith SG, Clarke D (2007) Melatonin and sleep disorders associated with intellectual disability: a clinical review. *J Intellect Disabil Res.* 51: 2–13.

van de Wouw E, Evenhuis HM, Echteld MA (2012) Prevalence, associated factors and treatment of sleep problems in adults with intellectual disability: a systematic review. *Res Dev Disabil.* 33(4): 1310–32.

CHAPTER 8

Women's Health Issues

Nyunt Nyunt Tin[1] & Julia Middleton[2,3]

[1]*Northamptonshire Healthcare NHS Foundation Trust, Northampton, UK*
[2]*Leicestershire Partnership NHS Trust, Leicester, UK*
[3]*Inclusion Healthcare Leicester, UK*

> For women with intellectual disability (ID), the expression and recognition of their mental distress may be complicated not only by their gender and ID but also by their communication needs and dependency on others and society at large.
>
> *O'Hara 2004*

Introduction

Women with ID are as likely to experience menstrual problems as the general population; however, such problems may present differently in women with ID and may not always be recognised due to difficulties in communication. The most frequently reported symptoms are pain, mood changes, anxiety related to bloodstained clothing or bedding, fatigue and heavy blood loss. These symptoms may present with behaviour and mental health problems in women with ID.

The behavioural and mental health problems related to the menstrual cycle that will be discussed in this chapter include:
- Premenstrual syndrome (PMS), including menstrual period-linked psychosis
- Problems related to childbearing years
- Polycystic ovary syndrome (PCOS)
- Catamenial epilepsy
- Perimenopausal problems

In the past, there has been a focus on menstrual suppression and elimination (therapeutic amenorrhoea) in women with ID to manage such problems; this, however, has legal and ethical concerns; therefore, there is a need for consensus guidelines in the area of management of behaviours and mental health problems

The Frith Prescribing Guidelines for People with Intellectual Disability, Third Edition.
Edited by Sabyasachi Bhaumik, David Branford, Mary Barrett and Satheesh Kumar Gangadharan.
© 2015 John Wiley & Sons, Ltd. Published 2015 by John Wiley & Sons, Ltd.

Table 8.1 Summary of steps in the assessment of menstrual cycle-related problems.

Full history, relevant physical examination and investigation
Exclude the presence of any other physical or psychiatric illness
Prospective rating of symptoms using agreed questionnaires or calendar sheets for at least two cycles
Check for symptom patterns and particularly the presence of an increase in symptoms in the premenstrual phase

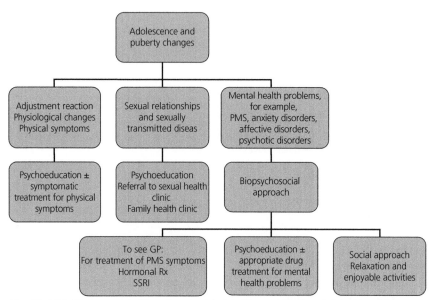

Algorithm 8.1 Management of keys issues related to the menstrual period during adolescence and puberty changes.

related to the menstrual period in women with ID. The main focus of this chapter therefore will be on the management of problems related to the menstrual period (Table 8.1 and Algorithm 8.1).

Definitions and aetiology

PMS can be broadly defined as the constellation of psychological and physical symptoms that recur regularly in the luteal phase of the menstrual cycle, remit for at least 1 week in the follicular phase and cause distress and functional impairment. The symptoms should be of at least moderate intensity and cause functional impairment. ICD-10 criteria include mild psychological symptoms, bloating, weight gain, breast tenderness, swelling, aches and pains, poor concentration, sleep disturbance and appetite change. Only one of these symptoms is required, but symptoms must be restricted to the luteal phase of the cycle, ceasing around menstruation. Severe symptoms that are predominantly dysphoric and cause severe impairment are referred to as premenstrual dysphoric disorder (DSM-IV).

There have been case reports of episodic psychosis linked to the menstrual period, which have the following characteristics: acute onset, short in duration with full recovery in between episodes and psychotic features (delusions, hallucinations and mood changes) recurring in rhythm with the menstrual cycle (Brockington).

The cause of PMS is poorly understood. Studies have shown that it is likely that several neurotransmitters may be involved, but there is no conclusive evidence. A genetic component, the GABA system, serotonergic system and endogenous opioids have all been linked to PMS.

Problems related to the childbearing years are no different from general population (see Table 8.1); however, additional issues in women with ID are ethical, legal (capacity to consent) and social issues that may have major impact on their mental well-being and behavioural issues. Key issues are capacity to consent, use of sterilisation, therapeutic amenorrhoea, developing parenting skills and mental health/distress consequent to a child being removed for fostering/adoption.

PCOS is a complex endocrine disorder presented with clinical symptoms: **hirsutism and acne** (due to excess androgens), **oligomenorrhoea or amenorrhoea and infertility** and **multiple cysts in the ovaries**. PCOS should be diagnosed if two or three of the criteria (highlighted in bold) are present, as long as other causes of menstrual disturbance and hyperandrogenism are excluded. Polycystic ovaries do not have to be present to make the diagnosis. Women with PCOS are at greater risk of developing long-term health problems such as type 2 diabetes, obesity and cardiovascular diseases. There are also reports of an association of developing PCOS in women taking sodium valproate for epilepsy during their young adulthood.

Catamenial epilepsy is a phenomenon of seizures worsening around the menstrual period. This exacerbation is thought to be a consequence of imbalance between the proconvulsant oestrogen and the anticonvulsant progesterone concentrations in the body during menstruation.

Perimenopausal issues refers to the phase of irregular menstrual activity that directly precedes menopause and is characterised by widely fluctuating hormone levels amidst a large-scale decline in circulating oestrogen. This phase in a woman's life is typically accompanied by physical discomfort including vasomotor symptoms, such as headaches, insomnia and hot flushes, as well as genital atrophy. Not surprisingly, studies suggest a significant increase in mood lability for women during this period. This phase may be difficult to recognise in women with ID especially when they have associated challenging behaviour, anxiety problems or communication difficulties.

Key issues through the life cycle

The onset of adolescence and puberty can be a particularly challenging time for young women with ID and their carers. Understanding and dealing with hormonal and bodily changes can prove difficult. Algorithm 8.1 highlights some of the key areas and their management.

Menstrual-related problems

Within the general population, it has been estimated that approximately 5% of menstruating women experience PMS as defined previously. It is estimated that up to 1.5 million women in the UK experience such severe symptoms that their quality of life and interpersonal relationships are greatly affected. At present, less than half of these women seek medical treatment.

Women with ID are similarly affected from menstrual period-related problems, but these may be further complicated by associated co-morbidities, for example, epilepsy treatment and communication difficulties. As yet there has been little research on their experiences or on the prevalence and appropriate management of problems related to the menstrual period in women in ID.

Key menstrual cycle issues specific to ID

- Most frequently reported symptoms are pain, mood changes, generally feeling unwell or tired and heavy blood loss.
- Women with severe/profound ID are more likely to have marked or severe period problems at some stage as compared to women with mild/moderate ID.
- Women with a coexisting physical impairment are more likely to experience marked or severe problems with their periods.
- In women with communication difficulties, symptoms may present in behaviours around the menstrual period.
- Younger women are more likely to experience menstrual problems as compared to women over the age of 35.
- Women with ID may experience menopause earlier than women in the general population.
- Women with Down syndrome are less likely to experience some problems such as feeling tired or unwell, heavy blood loss and sleep disturbance during their period than women without Down syndrome.
- The prevalence of epilepsy in PWID is higher than the general population and in women with ID, and this can be associated with catamenial epilepsy.
- There is a higher risk of developing PCOS in younger women with epilepsy who are prescribed sodium valproate.

Management

Table 8.2 illustrates common management approaches pertinent to menstrual cycle problems encountered at different life stages.

Psychiatric management is focused on a combination of treatment of mental illness and managing challenging behaviour, with an aim to improve their quality of life and well-being. Table 8.3 is for guidance only on the role of medications used

Table 8.2 Evidence base on roles of medication in managing menstrual period related problems.

Timeline	Key issues related to menstrual cycle at different stages of life	What to do/who to consult
Adolescence/ puberty changes	Adjustment reaction to pubertal changes (hormonal and physiological bodily changes)	Psychoeducation
	Mental and physical health problems related to onset of menarche and menstrual period, for example, PMS, dysmenorrhoea, acne, mastalgia, etc.	For physical symptoms – see Primary Care Physician\nFor mental health problems – Algorithm 8.1
	Sexual relationship and risk of sexually transmitted disease (STD)	Psychoeducation/sexual health clinic
	Contraception	To consult Primary Care Physician/family clinic
Childbearing age	Sexual relationship and risk of STD	Psychoeducation/sexual health clinic
	Premenstrual syndrome, dysmenorrhoea, acne, mastalgia, catamenial epilepsy	For physical symptoms – see Primary Care Physician\nEpilepsy – Primary Care Physician/neurologist/ ID psychiatrist
	Pregnancy and child birth, contraception, sterilisation, problems with medications crossing the placenta barrier and breast milk	See Primary Care Physician/family clinic
	Mental health problems: associated with puerperium, postnatal depression and puerperal psychosis	See psychiatrist
	Postnatal blues, stress and adjustment reaction related to parental responsibility and sleepless nights	Psychoeducation/Primary Care Physician
	Affective disorder, psychotic disorder and anxiety disorders	See relevant chapters of this guideline
Older age group (menopausal changes)	Age-related physical health – mobility problems, higher risk of osteoporosis after menopause	See Primary Care Physician for physical symptoms and menopausal symptoms
	Physical and mental health related to menopause	See relevant chapters of this guideline

in general in the management of menstrual period-related problems. Hormonal treatment and treatment for metabolic disorders are included in the table for information only as these areas of treatment are normally recommended by Primary Care Physicians and gynaecologists.

Table 8.3 Role of medication.

Problem	Medications used in management	Evidence
PMS	SSRI	There is increasing evidence that SSRIs and SNRIs are helpful in managing PMS and perimenopausal symptoms in general population In 31 randomised controlled trials that compared SSRIs with placebo, SSRIs were found to be effective for reducing the overall symptoms of PMS and also for reducing specific types of symptoms (psychological, physical and functional symptoms and irritability). SSRIs were usually taken for about 2 weeks before the start of the menstrual period. Both regimes appeared to be equally effective (Marjoribanks et al., 2013)
	SNRI	Efficacy and tolerability of premenstrual use of venlafaxine (flexible dose) in the treatment of premenstrual dysphoric disorder (Cohen et al., 2004)
	Anxiolytics – for example, buspirone	Buspirone has been shown to be superior to placebo but less effective than SSRIs. Compounds with affinity for serotonergic receptors in the treatment of premenstrual dysphoria: a comparison of buspirone, nefazodone and placebo (Landen et al., 2001)
	Hormone treatment: progesterone and progestogens in the luteal phase	Ten trials of progesterone and four of progestogens therapy for PMS were reviewed. All trials of progesterone therapy compared with placebo showed no difference, and although there was slight advantage of progestogens over placebo, meta-analysis showed no evidence for either (Ford et al., 2006)
	Combined oral contraceptive	Combination of drospirenone with ethyl estradiol (COC) may help treat severe premenstrual symptoms in women with premenstrual dysphoric disorder (PMDD). Cochrane Database Systematic Review in 2012 showed that the difference may not be clinically significant due to large placebo effect (Lopez et al., 2012)
	Danazol	Danazol helps with cyclical mastalgia during luteal phase but has androgenic side effects A randomised, placebo-controlled, crossover trial of danazol for the treatment of premenstrual syndrome (Hahn et al., 1995)
	Spironolactone	Given in luteal phase often helps with breast tenderness; bloating but need to monitor BP and electrolytes. Treatment of premenstrual syndrome by spironolactone: a double-blind, placebo-controlled study (Wang et al., 1995)

Condition	Treatment	Notes
Catamenial epilepsy	**Oestradiol patches and GnRH agonists**	Specialist prescription only
	Titrate up antiepileptic dose	
	Intermittent clobazam around menstrual period	In placebo controlled crossover study, intermittent use of clobazam versus placebo around the time of menstruation appeared to be superior to placebo (Feely, 1984)
	Spironolactone	
Polycystic ovary syndrome (**PCOS**)	**The 'old therapeutic tools'**	
	Oral contraceptives (OCP)	Therapeutic management should be individualised and not targeted on specific symptoms
	Anti-androgens	Currently available treatments for PCOS are not fully able to treat all the metabolic consequences (Bargiota and Diamanti-Kandarakis, 2012)
	The 'new therapeutic tools'	
	Insulin sensitisers: *metformin and thiazolidinediones*	
Perimenopausal symptoms	**Non-hormonal treatment**	
	SSRI	
	SNRI	SSRIs or SNRIs, compared to placebo, were found to be effective in reducing severe menopausal hot flushes among postmenopausal women (Freeman et al., 2011; Goodman, 2006; Joffe et al., 2014; Nelson et al., 2006)
	Hormonal treatment	HRT is currently the most effective treatment for vasomotor symptoms in postmenopausal women. Oestrogen remains the most effective treatment (Hickey et al., 2012)
	HRT	A Cochrane systematic review summarised the results of 24 placebo-controlled randomised trials that showed a clear beneficial effect with oestrogen replacement compared to placebo (Panay et al., 2013)

Illustrative case study 8.1

Susan, an 18-year-old young girl with mild ID and ASD, presented with history of episodic aggression and strange bizarre behaviour (sitting at the end of her bed, not moving for hours). She was first seen by a child psychiatrist 3 years ago, and during the assessment, a community nurse noticed she became quite strange and suspicious of other people including the nurse and family, episodically.

These bizarre episodes of behaviour were intermittent and lasted a few days. Susan's mother reported Susan had become very difficult and irritable, aggressive towards the family and also causing problems at school since she became a teenager. Family thought that was age-related rebellious behaviour. However, the behavioural problems had a clearly occurring intermittent pattern, and diary recording highlighted a clear relationship between her mental state and her menstrual period.

Intermittent treatment with progesterone prescribed by a gynaecologist, in combination with regular risperidone, produced a dramatic improvement in her mental state; progress was maintained with only occasional aggressive episodes coinciding with stressful situations.

Illustrative case study 8.2

Ruth is a 48-year-old woman with moderate/severe ID, plus challenging behaviour (stripping off naked, picking her skin deeply on face and breasts and lashing out at others). Carers who have known her for more than 20 years described these behaviours as long standing but now increasing in severity to an extent requiring physical intervention and also restricting her daily activities. They also report her periods have become very heavy, with clots.

Ruth was felt to be especially difficult to manage around her menstrual period, with risks to herself and aggression to others. Her Primary Care Physician referred to a gynaecologist and she was diagnosed with large uterine fibroids and prescribed a course of progesterone injections, which resulted in amenorrhoea for more than a year (an artificial menopause). Ruth's behaviour improved alongside this treatment, and her placement was maintained.

Discussion case study 8.3

Pamela is a 36-year-old woman with mild to moderate ID presenting with complex epilepsy and severe challenging behaviour (aggression towards others) who is living in a residential care home. Her seizures have been fairly well controlled for more than 10 years with current combination of sodium valproate 1 g BD and carbamazepine 600 mg BD. At present, she still has clusters of partial seizures, lasting up to 60 seconds, mainly occurring before her menstrual period.

Pamela attends her regular review with the local ID psychiatrist and complains of increasingly growing facial hair that she finds very distressing and wants treated. Carers report that for a number of years, she has been low in mood, quite irritable, argumentative and aggressive towards staff around her menstrual period. Her BMI is 32 and BP is 140/90 mmHg. She is compliant with her medication.
- What are the diagnostic possibilities?
- What management strategies could be tried?
- What is the role of medication in this case?

References

Bargiota A, Diamanti-Kandarakis E (2012) The effects of old, new and emerging medicines on metabolic aberrations in PCOS. *Therapeutic Advances in Endocrinology and Metabolism*, 3(1):27–47.

Cohen IS, Soares CN, Lyster AH, et al. (2004) Efficacy and tolerability of premenstrual use of venlafaxine (flexible dose) in the treatment of premenstrual dysphoric disorder. *Journal of Clinical Psychopharmacology*, 24:540–543.

Feely G (1984) Intermittent clobazam for catamenial epilepsy: tolerance avoided. *Journal of Neurology, Neurosurgery and Psychiatry*, 47:1279–1282.

Ford O, Lethaby A, Mol B, Roberts H (2006) Progesterone for premenstrual syndrome. *Cochrane Database of Systematic Review* (4):CD003415.

Freeman EW, Guthrie KA, Caan B, et al. (2011) Efficacy of escitalopram for hot flashes in healthy menopausal women: a randomized controlled trial. *JAMA*, 305(3):267–274.

Goodman A (2006) SNRI antidepressant reduces postmenopausal hot flashes. American Congress of Obstetricians and Gynecologists (ACOG) 59th Annual Clinical Meeting. Available at http://www.medscape.com/viewarticle/742234 (accessed on 14 February 2015).

Hahn PM, Van Vugt DA, Reid RL (1995) A randomized, placebo-controlled, crossover trial of danazol for the treatment of premenstrual syndrome. *Psychoneuroendocrinology*, 20:193–209.

Hickey M, Elliott J, Davison SL (2012) Hormone replacement therapy. *BMJ*, 344:e763.

Joffe H, Guthrie KA, LaCroix AZ, et al. (2014) Low-dose estradiol and the serotonin-norepinephrine reuptake inhibitor venlafaxine for vasomotor symptoms: a randomized clinical trial. *JAMA Internal Medicine*, 174(7):1058–1066.

Landen M, Eriksson O, Sundblad C, et al. (2001) Compounds with affinity for serotonergic receptors in the treatment of premenstrual dysphoria: a comparison of buspirone, nefazodone and placebo. *Psychopharmacology*, 155:292–298.

Lopez LM, Kaptein AA, Helmerhorst FM. (2012) Oral contraceptives containing drospirenone for premenstrual syndrome. *Cochrane Database Library* 2:CD006586.

Marjoribanks J, Brown J, O'Brien P, Wyatt K (2013) Selective serotonin reuptake inhibitors (SSRIs) for premenstrual syndrome. *Cochrane Database of Systematic Review* (6):CD001396.

Nelson HD, Vesco KK, Haney E, et al. (2006) Nonhormonal therapies for menopausal hot flashes systematic review and meta-analysis. *JAMA*, 295(17):2057–2071.

O'Hara J (2004) Mental health needs of women with learning disabilities: Services can be organised to meet the challenge. *Tizard Learning Disability Review*, 9(4):20–23.

Panay N, Hamoda H, Arya R, Savvas M (2013) The 2013 British Menopause Society & Women's Health Concern and recommendations on hormone replacement therapy. *Menopause International*, 19(2):59–68.

Wang M, Hammarbäck S, Lindhe BA, Bäckström T (1995) Treatment of premenstrual syndrome by spironolactone: a double-blind, placebo-controlled study. *Acta Obstetricia et Gynecologica Scandinavica*, 74:803–808.

Further reading

Brockington I (2005) Menstrual psychosis. *World Psychiatry*, 4(1):9–17.

Craig JJ (2007) Epilepsy and women. In: Sander JW, Walker MC, Smalls JE (eds.), *A practical guide to epilepsy – from cell to community*. West Hartford: International League Against Epilepsy, pp. 395–409.

Wyatt KM, Dimmock PW, Jones PW, O'Brien PMS (2001) Efficacy of progesterone and progestogens in management of premenstrual syndrome: systematic review. *British Medical Journal*, 323:1–8.

CHAPTER 9

Sexual Disorders

John Devapriam[1], Pancho Ghatak[2], Sabyasachi Bhaumik[1,3],
David Branford[4], Mary Barrett[1] & Sayeed Khan[1]

[1]*Leicestershire Partnership NHS Trust, Leicester, UK*
[2]*Partnerships in Care, Nottinghamshire, UK*
[3]*Department of Health Sciences, University of Leicester, Leicester, UK*
[4]*English Pharmacy Board, Royal Pharmaceutical Society, London, UK*

> It is with our passions, as it is with fire and water, they are good servants but bad masters.
>
> **Aesop**, *Greek slave & fable author (620–560 BC)*

Definition

The terms sexual offences and paraphilias are often used interchangeably in relevant literature, but these two terms need clarification. Only a proportion of sex offenders suffer from paraphilias. Also, not all people with a paraphilia are sex offenders. Frequently, they harbour deviant sexual fantasies and urges only, or their act does not cross the threshold of involving a non-consenting individual or a child.

In DSM-5, the term *paraphilia* is defined as any intense and persistent sexual interest other than sexual interest in genital stimulation or preparatory fondling with phenotypically normal, physically mature, consenting human partners. A *paraphilic disorder* is a paraphilia that has lasted for a period of at least 6 months and is causing distress or impairment to the individual or entails harm to others.

DSM-5 includes eight specific paraphilic disorders – voyeurism (spying on others in private activities), exhibitionism (exposing the genitals), frotteurism (touching or rubbing against a non-consenting individual), paedophilia (sexual focus on children), sexual masochism (undergoing humiliation, bondage or suffering), sexual sadism (inflicting humiliation, bondage or suffering), fetishism (using nonliving objects or having a highly specific focus on non-genital body parts) and transvestism (engaging in sexually arousing cross-dressing). They are relatively common, and some of them entail actions for their satisfaction that can be noxious or potentially harmful to others amounting to criminal offences. They, however, do not exhaust the list of possible paraphilic disorders.

The Frith Prescribing Guidelines for People with Intellectual Disability, Third Edition.
Edited by Sabyasachi Bhaumik, David Branford, Mary Barrett and Satheesh Kumar Gangadharan.
© 2015 John Wiley & Sons, Ltd. Published 2015 by John Wiley & Sons, Ltd.

Prevalence

The prevalence of ID in criminal populations remains a subject of considerable study and research. While many studies have highlighted ID as more prevalent among those who offend and those who offend sexually, no definitive figure is available about its prevalence. Studies conducted in different settings have produced differing prevalence rates of offenders and types of offending (Lindsay et al., 2007). A major factor in these studies has been the methodology to diagnose ID.

In their classical study, Walker and McCabe (1973) reviewed 331 men with ID detained under hospital orders for various offences and found high rates of fire raising (15%) and sexual offences (28%), when compared with other groups in the secure hospital sample. Holland and Persson (2010) studied a sample of 102 prisoners in Victoria, Australia and reported a prevalence rate of ID of less than 1.3% using the full Wechsler Adult Intelligence Scale (WAIS) by trained forensic psychologists. Hogue et al. (2006) studied three cohorts of individuals with ID across high secure, medium/low secure and community forensic services. There were no differences between these three cohorts in the rate of sexual disorders (34–50%).

Therefore, factors such as methodology employed to diagnose ID, varying inclusion criteria for studies, and studies conducted in a wide range of settings have made it difficult to reconcile the widely varying figures on the prevalence of ID in sexual offenders.

Aetiology

This seems to be multifactorial – neural, hormonal, genetic, psychological, developmental and cultural factors probably all play a part in paraphilic behaviours – making treatment complex. Testosterone, the main androgen produced by the testes, along with developing and maintaining male sexual characteristics, also controls sexuality, aggression, cognition and personality. Sexual fantasies, desire and behaviour are largely dependent on this hormone. It is clear that central serotonin metabolism also has a significant effect on sexual behaviour (Greenberg & Bradford, 1997). Animal research has shown that when brain serotonin levels are decreased, there is an increase in sexual drive and mounting behaviour. These behaviours are likewise reduced when serotonin levels in the brain are increased.

Empirical studies have shown an increased prevalence of various factors including history of sexual abuse in childhood, attachment difficulties, social incompetence, emotional dysregulation and disinhibition caused by empathy deficits in people with paedophilia and other paraphilias (Yakeley & Wood, 2014).

Treatment of sexual offenders

The remit of this chapter is pharmacological treatment options only; however, it should be emphasised that the mainstay of treatment in sexual offenders is psychological therapy, which offers the prospect of long-lasting change

(Yakeley & Wood, 2014). The different modalities found beneficial in this group include cognitive–behavioural therapy (social skills training, cognitive restructuring, development of victim empathy and imaginal desensitisation) and relapse prevention therapy (focused on dynamic factors such as intimacy, attachment, emotion regulation and impulsivity). Treatment approaches such as the sex offenders treatment programme (SOTP) are generally available to average ability offenders (those with IQ above 80), and an adapted programme has been developed to suit the treatment needs of offenders with intellectual disability (ASOTP). Treatment can be delivered in community settings or in institutions (prisons and specialist hospitals) and is usually in the form of group therapy. It is suggested that readers refer to appropriate texts on psychological therapies for sexual offenders with ID.

Evidence base for the use of psychotropic medications

Though psychotropic medications have been in use for some time, the level of evidence is very poor (case reports, small sample size, etc.), and the efficacy has not been shown in any randomised controlled trials.

Mood stabilisers: Lithium carbonate and anticonvulsants have been in use for years, but they have shown no efficacy in the absence of a concurrent bipolar disorder.

Antipsychotics: Drugs like benperidol, chlorpromazine, haloperidol and risperidone have been used. No significant differences were evident in comparison studies. Apart from rare cases, where paraphilic behaviours have been associated with delusional beliefs of schizophrenia, no clear efficacy has been found with the use of antipsychotics.

Selective serotonin reuptake inhibitors (SSRIs): There has been significant research evidence on the efficacy of SSRIs. Exhibitionism, compulsive masturbation and paedophilia have all shown improvement following SSRI treatment:
- Sertraline reduces deviant sexual behaviours – but it does not affect, and sometimes even improves, normal sexuality (Bradford et al., 1995; Bradford, 2000).
- SSRIs prescribed to individuals between 12 and 18 years could prevent acting out of deviant fantasies and behaviour (Bradford & Fedoroff, 2006).
- SSRIs may be particularly useful in paraphilias associated with OCD and depression and in individuals with a strong compulsive element to their sexual urges that they find difficult to resist.

Anti-androgens
1 *Medroxyprogesterone acetate (MPA)*:
   - Reduces plasma testosterone and availability of free testosterone.
   - In spite of evidence of efficacy, because of serious side effects (weight gain, hypertension, adrenal suppression, thromboembolism, etc.), use of MPA has been abandoned in Europe.

2 *Cyproterone acetate (CPA):*
- A synthetic steroid resembling progesterone – acts as both progestogen and anti-androgen.
- Evidence is based on case reports, open and controlled studies, for efficacy, dosage and duration of treatment
- Indication: See levels 3 and 4 of Algorithm 9.1.
- Many authors recommend 3–5 years of treatment. Treatment effects are completely reversible in 1–2 months following discontinuation of treatment.
- Side effects: Sleep disorders, depression, osteoporosis, thromboembolism, hypertension, renal and cardiac dysfunction, hepatocellular dysfunction, gynaecomastia (rarely leading to galactorrhoea and benign breast nodules), etc. Fatality has been reported especially when CPA has been prescribed at more than 200–300 mg/day and after several months of treatment. However, serious hepatotoxicity is uncommon, <1%.
- Pretreatment investigations: Liver functions tests, full blood count, ECG, fasting glucose, blood pressure, weight, calcium and phosphate levels, U&Es, bone mineral density, testosterone, FSH, LH and plasma prolactin levels.
- Monitoring: Blood counts, liver function tests and adrenocortical function.
- Contraindications for CPA: Non-consent; puberty not completed; liver disease; diabetes mellitus; severe hypertension; carcinoma (apart from prostate carcinoma); meningioma; pregnancy or breastfeeding; previous thromboembolic disease; cardiac, pituitary or adrenal disorders; tuberculosis; epilepsy; psychosis; etc.

3 *Gonadotrophin-releasing hormone (GnRH) analogues:*
- Because of poor treatment compliance with CPA, there has been a need for an effective group of medications with lesser side effects.
- Bilateral orchidectomy is associated with a significant reduction of circulating androgen level, and this has been associated with lowest rates of recidivism among all forms of treatment. This had led to more research in GnRH analogues.
- GnRH analogues stimulate the pituitary to release LH → transient increase in serum testosterone → continued administration → down-regulation of GnRH receptors → reduction of LH, FSH and testosterone to castration levels within 2–4 weeks.
- Efficacy observed was very high in open studies. A reduction of deviant sexual fantasies and behaviour was observed.
- Of the GnRH analogues, only triptorelin is indicated in the treatment of male hypersexuality with severe sexual deviation and will be discussed here.

Triptorelin
- Synthetic decapeptide agonist, analogue of GnRH.
- Indication: See level 5 of Algorithm 9.1.
- Dose: By intramuscular injection, 11.25 mg every 3 months (level 5 of Algorithm 9.1).

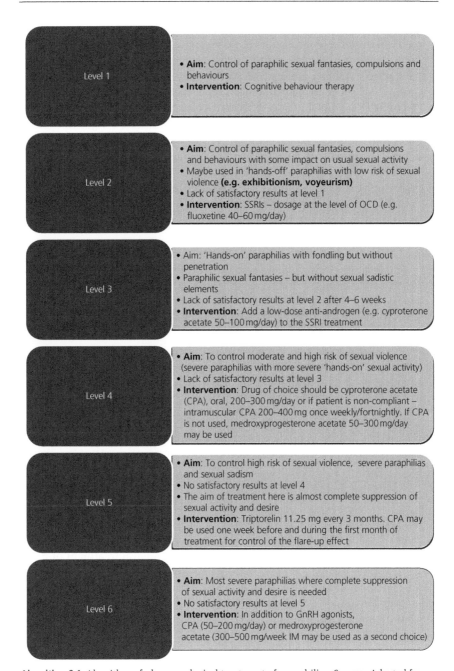

Level 1
- **Aim**: Control of paraphilic sexual fantasies, compulsions and behaviours
- **Intervention**: Cognitive behaviour therapy

Level 2
- **Aim**: Control of paraphilic sexual fantasies, compulsions and behaviours with some impact on usual sexual activity
- Maybe used in 'hands-off' paraphilias with low risk of sexual violence **(e.g. exhibitionism, voyeurism)**
- Lack of satisfactory results at level 1
- **Intervention**: SSRIs – dosage at the level of OCD (e.g. fluoxetine 40–60 mg/day)

Level 3
- Aim: 'Hands-on' paraphilias with fondling but without penetration
- Paraphilic sexual fantasies – but without sexual sadistic elements
- Lack of satisfactory results at level 2 after 4–6 weeks
- **Intervention**: Add a low-dose anti-androgen (e.g. cyproterone acetate 50–100 mg/day) to the SSRI treatment

Level 4
- **Aim**: To control moderate and high risk of sexual violence (severe paraphilias with more severe 'hands-on' sexual activity)
- Lack of satisfactory results at level 3
- **Intervention**: Drug of choice should be cyproterone acetate (CPA), oral, 200–300 mg/day or if patient is non-compliant – intramuscular CPA 200–400 mg once weekly/fortnightly. If CPA is not used, medroxyprogesterone acetate 50–300 mg/day may be used

Level 5
- **Aim**: To control high risk of sexual violence, severe paraphilias and sexual sadism
- No satisfactory results at level 4
- The aim of treatment here is almost complete suppression of sexual activity and desire
- **Intervention**: Triptorelin 11.25 mg every 3 months. CPA may be used one week before and during the first month of treatment for control of the flare-up effect

Level 6
- **Aim**: Most severe paraphilias where complete suppression of sexual activity and desire is needed
- No satisfactory results at level 5
- **Intervention**: In addition to GnRH agonists, CPA (50–200 mg/day) or medroxyprogesterone acetate (300–500 mg/week IM may be used as a second choice)

Algorithm 9.1 Algorithm of pharmacological treatment of paraphilias. Source: Adapted from Thibaut et al. (2010). © Informa Healthcare.

- Duration of treatment remains a matter of debate. Thibaut et al. feel that a minimum duration of 3 years is necessary to attain a stable state and, for some patients, lifelong treatment might be necessary.
- Side effects: Decrease in trabecular bone density, hypertension, musculoskeletal pain or weakness, changes in scalp and body hair, facial oedema and oedema of extremities and mood changes including depression.
- Pretreatment workup: Physical examination including weight and blood pressure. Plasma testosterone, FSH, LH, blood glucose, calcium and phosphate, lipid profile, renal function and ECG must be undertaken. For patients with risk of osteoporosis, bone mineral density should be checked. Careful monitoring needs to continue for emotional and mood problems (every 1–3 months), blood parameters every 6 months and bone mineral density every year for patients with risk of osteoporosis.

Illustrative case study 9.1

Sam, a 26-year-old male with mild ID, was admitted to a low secure unit for repeated paedophilic activities (non-penetrative acts) and with vivid paedophiliac sexual fantasies. There was no element of violence in his fantasies and activities. He underwent a Sexual Offenders Treatment Programme (CBT based), but there was only mild reduction to his sexual fantasies following this.

The multidisciplinary team then reviewed his treatment and offered him CPA at a dose of 50 mg/day. Sam gave informed consent to the treatment. He reported reduction of sexual fantasies after about six months of treatment. After about a year, his CBT programme was repeated, and his response to the psychotherapy was much better this time (CPA was maintained alongside). At the end of the cycle, he reported that he does not get paraphilic fantasies any more. There was no report of offence parallel behaviour on the ward and during escorted leave to the community. It was felt that he could now be moved to a locked rehabilitation unit and this was facilitated. All the recommended monitoring for CPA continued throughout his stay.

Florence Thibaut et al. (2010) published 'The World Federation of Societies of Biological Psychiatry (WFSBP) guidelines for the biological treatment of paraphilias'. This evaluated the role of pharmacotherapy in the treatment and management of paraphilias. The authors used an extensive literature search in the English language on MEDLINE/PubMed as well as other published reviews. An algorithm was proposed with six levels of treatment for different categories of paraphilias.

Though these guidelines are not specific for patients with ID, they can provide valuable clinical options, in addition to psychological therapy, in treating sexual disorders in patients with ID employing the usual clinical considerations and cautions applicable in this patient group.

Discussion case study 9.2

Richard is a 55-year-old man with mild ID and epilepsy who had been a resident in a long-stay ID facility since his teens. He is an informal patient and was described as a 'model' resident on the ward, helpful to staff and visitors, with no behavioural concerns reported in that environment. Richard attends the on-site sheltered workshop daily where he earns a therapeutic wage. He likes to go into the local town independently where he will spend his wages on sweets and comics. During these trips, he has repeatedly approached young adolescent boys and offered them sweets and comics in exchange for becoming his friend. On a number of these occasions, he has been reported to the police and charges brought; however, he has never been successfully prosecuted. Whenever there is an impending court appearance, Richard acknowledges his behaviour and appears keen to engage in treatment, but afterwards, he quickly disengages. Richard now has a reputation in the local community for this behaviour and has been physically assaulted on three separate occasions as a consequence. He however remains insistent on continuing his usual outings unaccompanied.

Questions:
- What are the risks?
- How would you manage this situation?
- Which agencies should be involved and what is their role?

References

Bradford, J. M. W. (2000). The treatment of sexual deviation using a pharmacological approach. *Journal of Sex Research*, 3, 248–257.

Bradford, J. M. W. & Fedoroff, P. (2006). Pharmacological treatment of the juvenile sex offender. In H. E. Barbaree & W. L. Marshall (Eds.). *The juvenile sex offender* (2nd ed.) (pp. 358–383). New York: Guilford.

Bradford, J. M. W., Greenberg, D. M., Gojer, J. J., Martindale, J. J. & Goldberg, M. (1995). Sertraline in the treatment of pedophilia – an open labelled study. Paper presented at the Annual American Psychiatric Association Congress, Miami, FL, May.

Greenberg, D. M. & Bradford, J. M. W. (1997). Treatment of the paraphilic disorders: a review of the role of the selective serotonin reuptake inhibitors. *Sexual Abuse*, 9, 349–361.

Hogue, T., Steptoe, L., Taylor, J. L., et al. (2006). A comparison of offenders with intellectual disability across three levels of security. *Criminal Behaviour and Mental Health*, 16, 13–28.

Holland, S. & Persson, P. (2010). Intellectual disability in the Victorian prison system: characteristics of prisoners with an intellectual disability released from prison in 2003–2006. *Psychology Crime and Law*, 17(1), 25–41.

Lindsay, W. R., Hastings, R. P., Griffiths, D. M. & Hayes, S. C. (2007). Trends and challenges in forensic research on offenders with intellectual disability. *Journal of Intellectual and Developmental Disability*, 32, 55–61.

Thibaut, F., de la Barra, F., Gordon, H., Cosyns, P., Bradford, J. M. W. & the WFSBP Task Force on Sexual Disorders (2010). The World Federation of Societies of Biological Psychiatry (WFSBP) guidelines for the biological treatment of paraphilias. *The World Journal of Biological Psychiatry*, 11, 604–655.

Walker, N. & McCabe, S. (1973). *Crime and insanity in England* (Vol. 2). Edinburgh: Edinburgh University Press.

Yakeley, J. & Wood, H. (2014). Paraphilias and paraphilic disorder: diagnosis, assessment and management. *Advances in Psychiatric Treatment*, 20, 202–213.

Further reading

Bradford, J. M. W. (1985). Organic treatments for the male sexual offender. *Behavioural Sciences & the Law*, 3, 355–375.

Bradford, J. M. W. & Kaye, N. S. (1999). Pharmacological treatment of sexual offenders. *American Academy of Psychiatry and Law Newsletter*, 24, 16–17.

Clarke, D. (1989). Antilibidinal drugs and mental retardation: a review. *Medicine, Science and the Law*, 29(2), 136–146.

Craig, L. A., Lindsay, W. R. & Browne, K. D. (2010). *Assessment and treatment of sexual offenders with intellectual disabilities: a handbook*. Chichester: John Wiley & Sons, Ltd.

Gordon, H. & Grubin, D. (2004). Psychiatric aspects of the assessment and treatment of sex offenders. *Advances in Psychiatric Treatment*, 10, 73–80.

Lindsay, W. R. (2009). *The treatment of sex offenders with developmental disabilities: a practice workbook*. Hoboken, NJ: John Wiley & Sons, Inc.

Lindsay, W. R., Hastings, R. P. & Beech, A. R. (2011). Forensic research in offenders with intellectual & developmental disabilities 1: prevalence and risk assessment. Special issue: Forensic research in offenders with intellectual & developmental disabilities Part 1. *Psychology, Crime & Law*, 17(1), 3–7.

Rosler, A. & Witztum, E. (1998). Treatment of men with paraphilia with a long-acting analogue of gonadotropin-releasing hormone. *New England Journal of Medicine*, 338, 416–422.

CHAPTER 10

Autism Spectrum Disorders

Mary Barrett[1] & Elspeth Bradley[2,3]

[1]*Leicestershire Partnership NHS Trust, Leicester, UK*
[2]*Surrey Place Centre, Toronto, Ontario, Canada*
[3]*Department of Psychiatry, University of Toronto, Toronto, Ontario, Canada*

Autism is a life-long, often devastating, disorder that profoundly affects almost every aspect of an individual's functioning.

Howlin, 1997

Definition

Autism spectrum disorders (ASD) are a group of severe developmental and neuropsychiatric disorders usually apparent by the age of 3 years. Autism was first described by Leo Kanner in 1943 and Asperger syndrome by Hans Asperger a year later in 1944; however, wider awareness of the conditions began with the work of Lorna Wing. From her field research, Wing later drew up a triad of behavioural criteria for the diagnosis of autistic disorder. These impairments are found in people with ASD throughout the range of intelligence and in all the clinical subtypes.

Wing's triad of impairments:

- Qualitative impairment in reciprocal social interaction
- Qualitative impairment in verbal and non-verbal communication and in imaginative activity
- Markedly restricted repertoire of activities and interests

Clinical presentation

Table 10.1 lists the common core characteristics of ASD. All the individual characteristics are variable in degree and nature in any given person; however, abnormalities should be present from each domain for a diagnosis to be made.

The Frith Prescribing Guidelines for People with Intellectual Disability, Third Edition.
Edited by Sabyasachi Bhaumik, David Branford, Mary Barrett and Satheesh Kumar Gangadharan.
© 2015 John Wiley & Sons, Ltd. Published 2015 by John Wiley & Sons, Ltd.

Although a diagnosis of ASD requires the presence of the core triad of impairments, the clinical presentation of ASD varies from individual to individual and may alter in any given person over time. One key factor affecting this variability is intelligence level (IQ). Although ASD may present with a variety of features at any intellectual level, certain pictures are more common with particular IQ levels and different diagnostic subcategories (Figure 10.1).

Table 10.1 Common core characteristics of ASD.

Domain	Key features
Social impairment	Difficulty with social cues affecting reciprocal social interaction, joint interactive play and joint attention behaviour
	Failure to recognise emotional cues, resulting in inappropriate responses to distress in others, reflecting a wider lack of empathy
Communication impairment	Both verbal and non-verbal spheres of language are affected
	Impairment of social communication, including two-way interactions, is key
	Expressive function is more affected that receptive language
	Both symbolic and pragmatic language abnormalities occur, including echolalia, abnormal prosody, pronoun reversal and lack of variation in the quality of speech
Impairment of imagination and behaviour	Interests and activities are limited to a few circumscribed themes, with a lack of spontaneity, imaginativeness and creativity
	Activities are typically repetitive and stereotyped
	Interest in a part of, or non-functional element of an object, for example, texture rather than the whole
	Compulsive routines and unusual attachments, which can result in large collections and storage problems
	Any unexpected change may result in distress, agitation and/or aggression

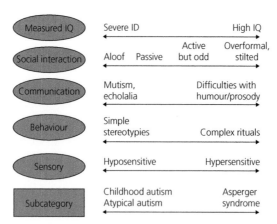

Figure 10.1 Presentation of ASD across the IQ spectrum.

In addition to the core characteristics, there are a number of other key features and other conditions commonly associated with ASD, including sensory sensitivities and motor abnormalities. Common problems include abnormal perceptions, particularly in hearing and vision, which can lead to sensory overload, and motor dysfunction presenting as hand flapping, bouncing up and down and/or gyration.

Lack of awareness and internal monitoring of time and space can also cause major difficulties, rendering the person unable to think in a sequential framework and thus to understand and predict the world.

These factors all need to be taken into account when assessing a person with an ASD, and indeed, some of these factors may prove a more significant management challenge than the core features themselves. Figure 10.2 illustrates the complexity of the clinical picture.

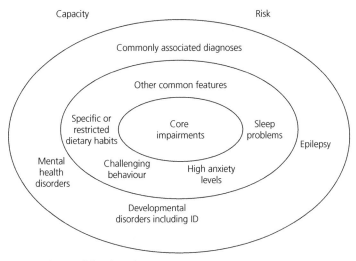

Figure 10.2 Complexity of the clinical picture in ASD.

Prevalence

Brugha et al. (2012) found that:
- The overall prevalence of autism in England is estimated at 1.1%
- The prevalence is higher in men than women (2 vs. 0.3%)

Specifically within the ID population, the study found that:
- The prevalence of autism in adults with ID living in communal care establishments was 31% and in private households was 35.4%
- The prevalence of autism increased with increasing degree of ID
- The prevalence of autism increased with decreasing verbal IQ
- Sex differences were less marked in adults with ID (60% men vs. 43% women with profound ID)

Management

The management of ASD begins with accurate recognition and diagnosis of both the core condition and any associated features. Given the high prevalence rates, it is vital that clinicians are 'autism aware' whenever they are assessing someone with an ID.

Illustrative case study 10.1

A 52-year-old man with moderate ID and a long-standing history of challenging behaviour was re-referred to the psychiatrist in the community team, after becoming increasingly aggressive in the residential home where he lived. The psychiatrist visited the gentleman at home and noted that common triggers for aggressive outbursts included the day centre bus being late, other residents moving the ornaments around in the communal lounge and the hand dryer in the bathroom being switched on. On questioning, it further became apparent that the man rarely made eye contact, only voluntarily interacted with staff when he wanted a hot drink and much of his speech consisted of stock phrases, for example, 'It's raining today', which were usually said out of context.

The psychiatrist completed a standardised interview schedule with the staff and the man's mother and a member of the community ID team carried out a series of behavioural observations in the residential home and the day centre. Following this, a diagnosis of autism was made and an intervention package designed, including staff education around ASD, input from a speech and language therapist to develop a communication passport and visual timetable, sensory assessment and sensory integration work by an occupational therapist and negotiation with the transport service to allow the gentleman to be picked up first to avoid any unnecessary delays.

Role of medication

At present, there is no 'cure' for ASD and its core characteristics. Clinical focus is centred on the management of consequent behavioural issues and maximising functioning, rather than the primary condition itself. Key management approaches include appropriate educational provision, environmental adaptations, behavioural interventions, family/carer support and education around the condition. There is also increasing emphasis on the value of early intervention work.

Medication treatment has a limited role to play in the treatment of ASD per se and should only be considered:

1 As part of an overall management plan.

2 If environmental, behavioural and psychological strategies have proved insufficient.

3 If there is a significant impact on the functioning of the person/those around them. This includes potential or actual risks arising from the behaviour.

Repetitive behaviours are common, including stereotypies and rituals. These behaviours may have a significant impact on the functioning of the individual and/or those around them. Interruption of such behaviours may cause great distress, in turn resulting in disturbed behaviour. Stereotypies are likely mediated by dopamine and therefore respond best to medications such as risperidone, while rituals and other obsessive behaviours are mediated by serotonin and therefore may respond better to SSRIs.

Medication treatment of co-morbid mental health issues should be considered as for any individual, irrespective of the diagnosis of ASD. This notwithstanding, the propensity for anxiety and mood disorders in people with ASD should be noted here, including the fact that the presentation may be atypical for example an increase in stereotypies or aggression/self-injury. A trial of medication may be warranted if an underlying mental health disorder is suspected.

Catatonia, occurring in the context of ASD, has been variously reported in the literature, including by Lorna Wing. Treatment with lorazepam – in some cases to high doses – has been reported as being of benefit in individual cases; however, formal trial data is lacking.

Aggression and self-injurious behaviour (SIB) may also warrant a trial of medication treatment in their own right, as a last resort. Medication should only be considered as part of an overall treatment strategy based on functional analysis, with contingency management as the primary objective of the intervention. Risk assessment will be a key part of any consideration to prescribe, and medication should be regularly reviewed, with the aim of limiting both use and duration of treatment to a minimum.

Choosing a medication

The evidence base for medication in ASD remains limited; however, the available data is summarised in Table 10.2.

When choosing a medication, it is vital to be clear what symptom(s) you are targeting. Algorithm 10.1 summarises the key domains that may be targeted in a person with ASD. It is important to remember that a person may have symptoms in several domains, and treatment choices and order should be tailored accordingly. This is illustrated in case study 10.2.

Table 10.2 Evidence base for medication treatment in ASD.

Medication	Overview of evidence from specific medication trials of benefits in autism
Antipsychotics	
Risperidone Usual doses of 1–2 mg daily	Cochrane review (Cochrane, 2010) identified three randomised controlled trials. Meta-analysis was possible for three outcomes. Some evidence of benefit for irritability, repetition and social withdrawal. These must, however, be considered against adverse effects, most prominently weight gain
	Controlled trials in children have suggested that given the adverse events observed and lack of a clear benefit with regard to core autism symptoms, risperidone should be reserved for treatment of moderate to severe behavioural problems associated with autism
Aripiprazole Starting dose of aripiprazole for paediatric patients with autism is 2 mg/day, increasing to 5 mg/day and then subsequently increased to 10 or 15 mg/day as needed	The US Food and Drug Administration (FDA) has approved an expanded indication for the oral formulation of aripiprazole orally disintegrating tablets and oral solution, for the treatment of irritability associated with ASD, as part of a total paediatric treatment programme that includes psychological, educational and social interventions
	The approval was based on data from two, 8-week, randomised, placebo-controlled multicentre studies
	For both studies, the most frequently reported aripiprazole-related adverse events (incidence >10%, twice that of placebo) were sedation (21 vs. 4%), fatigue (17 vs. 2%), vomiting (14 vs. 7%), somnolence (10 vs. 4%) and tremor (10 vs. 0%)
	The most common reasons for discontinuation were sedation, drooling, tremor, vomiting and extrapyramidal disorder. Clinically significant weight gain (>7 lb) occurred in 26% of patients receiving aripiprazole compared with 7% of those receiving placebo (mean gain, 1.6 vs. 0.4 kg, respectively)
Olanzapine	Very limited evidence base. Small trials have shown benefit in alleviating some behavioural symptoms (irritability, hyperactivity/noncompliance and lethargy/withdrawal) associated with autism. Concerns over weight gain and metabolic side effects
Haloperidol Usual doses of 1–2 mg daily	Licensed for short-term adjunctive management of psychomotor agitation, excitement and violent and dangerous impulsive behaviour
	Haloperidol has been found effective for reducing behavioural symptoms such as hyperactivity, aggression, stereotypies, affective lability and tantrums, but not for treating the core symptoms of autism
	Haloperidol is associated with a high incidence of tardive and withdrawal dyskinesias, and clinical use is significantly limited due to these side effects
Quetiapine	A number of very small open trials using low doses have shown limited short-term effects on symptoms such as aggression
Antidepressants	
SSRIs	A Cochrane review (2013) found nine trials, involving 320 people, which evaluated four SSRIs: fluoxetine, fluvoxamine, fenfluramine and citalopram. Five studies included only children and four studies included only adults. One trial enrolled 149 children, but the other trials were much smaller. There was no evidence to support the use of SSRIs to treat autism in children, and limited evidence, which was felt not yet sufficiently robust, to suggest effectiveness of SSRIs in adults with autism. It was noted that treatment with an SSRI may cause side effects. The authors concluded that decisions about the use of SSRIs for established clinical indications that may co-occur with autism, such as obsessive–compulsive disorder and depression in adults or children, and anxiety in adults, should be made on a case-by-case basis

Other antidepressants	An open, retrospective clinical study with venlafaxine evaluated its effect on core symptoms of autism as well as associated features of ADHD. Six of 10 completers were judged to be sustained treatment responders at low doses (mean, 24.37 mg/day; range, 6.25–50 mg/day) and tolerated the medication well. Improvement was noted in repetitive behaviours and restricted interests, social deficits, communication and language function, inattention and hyperactivity
	Clomipramine has been reported as causing improvements in social interaction, aggression and repetitive thoughts and behaviour in four of five young adults with autism following open-label treatment
	In a double-blind crossover study, clomipramine was found superior to desipramine and placebo in controlling symptoms of autism and anger as well as improving symptoms of hyperactivity in a group of children and adolescents
	Additional studies, including an open-label trial involving 35 adults, have supported a role for clomipramine in the amelioration of repetitive behaviour and aggression. However, an open-label investigation utilising clomipramine in the treatment of eight children with pervasive developmental disorders (PDDs) described clinical worsening in seven and poor tolerance of the medication
	Very small trials of mirtazapine in 26 children and adults showed only modest effect
	One trial of duloxetine and agomelatine failed to show any additional benefits
Stimulants	Depending on the research methods, studies estimate attention deficit hyperactivity disorder (ADHD) occurs in 14–80% of this patient population and may be even more troublesome than the core symptoms of autism
Methylphenidate	The 2005 trial conducted by the Research Units on Paediatric Psychopharmacology (RUPP) Autism Network showed that immediate-release methylphenidate (IR-MPH) decreased hyperactivity, improved attention span and possibly enhanced communication skills in ASD and ADHD children. However, IR-MPH also was associated with an increased risk for irritability and corresponding social withdrawal, and response rates varied widely
	Further studies have suggested that there appears to be a dose-dependent improvement in hyperactivity symptoms in children with ASD and co-morbid ADHD
Clonidine	The evidence to support clonidine remains mixed
	In very small trials, it has been shown to be effective in reducing impulsivity, inattention and hyperactivity, as well as in serving as a sedative in children with autism and sleep disorders. One trial using transdermal clonidine was limited by skin irritation
Antiepileptics	
Valproate	Studies show improvements in repetitive behaviours, social relatedness, aggression and mood lability; however, the responders all had abnormal EEGs. Another small double-blind study showed benefit with repetitive behaviours
Lamotrigine	Initial studies suggested improvement in social engagement, attention and alertness, but later studies failed to demonstrate this
Other antiepileptics	Despite its widespread use, there are no studies of carbamazepine. Small studies of levetiracetam suggested benefit to hyperactivity and impulsiveness. Studies of topiramate as an add-on for weight loss showed worsening of agitation and irritability

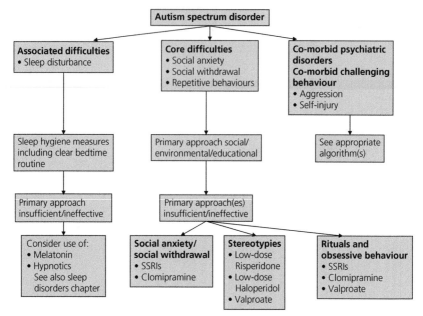

Algorithm 10.1 Medication treatment in ASD.

Illustrative case study 10.2

> A 25-year-old lady with severe ID and known ASD started to self-injure, repetitively hitting the right side of her head with her fist, to the extent of causing tissue damage. Physical examination revealed evidence of earwax build-up in the right ear canal, which was successfully treated. After treatment, however, the behaviour continued and no further physical, psychiatric or environmental cause could be identified. Detailed observation revealed that attempts by staff to stop the behaviour led to the lady becoming increasingly distressed and hitting her head with renewed vigour, and it was concluded that the behaviour now appeared compulsive in nature. A behavioural programme was commenced that had limited effect, so an SSRI was trialled. This combination of strategies produced significant lessening of the behaviour, which allowed the tissue damage to heal.

Discussion case study 10.3

> Brian, a 72-year-old man with mild ID and ASD living in residential care becomes increasingly reluctant to go out of the house and participate in his usual day care programme. He insists on spending increasing periods of time in his room arranging his collection of newspapers and magazines and becomes very agitated if staff attempt to engage with him during this process. Over a period of weeks, he becomes increasingly nocturnal, not going to sleep until 3–4 AM and then staying in bed all morning. At this point, Brian is referred by his social worker to the community ID team for assessment and input.
> - What are the diagnostic possibilities?
> - What management strategies could be tried?
> - What is the role of medication in this case?

References

Brugha T, Cooper SA, McManus S, et al. (2012). Extending the 2007 adult psychiatric morbidity survey. http://www.hscic.gov.uk/catalogue/PUB05061/esti-prev-auti-ext-07-psyc-morb-surv-rep.pdf (accessed 11 February 2015).

Cochrane (2010). Risperidone for autism spectrum disorder. http://www.cochrane.org/CD005040/BEHAV_risperidone-for-autism-spectrum-disorder (accessed 11 February 2015).

Cochrane (2013). Selective serotonin reuptake inhibitors (SSRIs) for autism spectrum disorders (ASD). http://onlinelibrary.wiley.com/doi/10.1002/14651858.CD004677.pub3/full (accessed 16 February 2015).

Howlin P (1997). *Autism, preparing for adulthood*. London: Routledge.

Further reading

NHS Information Centre for Health and Social Care (2012). Estimating the prevalence of autism spectrum conditions in adults: Extending the 2007 adult psychiatric morbidity survey. http://www.ic.nhs.uk/pubs/autism11 (accessed 7 January 2015).

NICE (2011a). Autism diagnosis in children and young people: Recognition, referral and diagnosis of children and young people on the autism spectrum (CG 128). http://www.nice.org.uk/CG128 (accessed 7 January 2015).

NICE (2011b). Autism: Recognition, referral, diagnosis and management of adults on the autism spectrum. http://www.nice.org.uk/guidance/cg142 (accessed 11 February 2015).

CHAPTER 11

Attention Deficit Hyperactivity Disorder

Karen Bretherton
Leicestershire Partnership NHS Trust, Leicester, UK

> Having ADHD is like having a powerful race car for a brain, which is inappropriately equipped with bicycle brakes.
>
> *Kimberley Faith Wood*

Definition

Attention deficit hyperactivity disorder (ADHD) is a heterogeneous condition presenting with hyperactivity, impulsivity and inattention that is pervasive, commences in childhood, impairs functioning and cannot be attributed to the developmental level.

Diagnostic criteria

DSM-5 uses the diagnostic term ADHD; however, ICD-10 uses the term hyperkinetic disorder. The DSM diagnosis allows for subtypes to be diagnosed, namely, predominantly inattentive, predominantly hyperactive/impulsive and combined. ICD-10 requires the full combined criteria to be met (Table 11.1).

The Diagnostic Criteria for Psychiatric Disorders for Use with Adults with Learning Disabilities/Mental Retardation (DC-LD) adds helpful clarity to applying these diagnostic criteria to adults with intellectual disability (ID). To summarise the criteria, the DC-LD states, 'In adults with learning disability the disorder may be overlooked because the combination of poor attention, impulsive, disorganised behaviour, and difficulty in initiating and maintaining purposeful behaviour is

The Frith Prescribing Guidelines for People with Intellectual Disability, Third Edition.
Edited by Sabyasachi Bhaumik, David Branford, Mary Barrett and Satheesh Kumar Gangadharan.
© 2015 John Wiley & Sons, Ltd. Published 2015 by John Wiley & Sons, Ltd.

Table 11.1 Diagnostic criteria.

	DSM-5	ICD-10
Age of onset	Symptoms present prior to age 12	Before the age of 7
Cardinal features	Either inattention or hyperactivity	Both inattention and hyperactivity
	Symptoms present in two or more settings	Present in two or more settings
	Evidence that the symptoms impair functioning or reduce quality of social, school or work skills	Evidence of impairment from the symptoms in social, academic or occupational functioning
	Symptoms do not occur only during course of psychosis or other mental health disorder	Symptoms do not occur exclusively during pervasive developmental disorder, psychosis or other mental health disorders
	Symptoms persisted for more than 6 months and not attributed to developmental level	Symptoms persisted for more than 6 months and not attributed to developmental level
Presence of	Six or more inattentive symptoms for children up to age 16 or five or more symptoms for those over age 17	Six or more inattentive symptoms, for example
	Difficulty in sustaining attention	Poor attention in school work or work
	Fails to give close attention to details	Fails to sustain attention in tasks or play
	Does not seem to be listening when spoken to directly	Appears not to listen when spoken to directly
	Does not follow through on instructions	Does not follow through on instructions or tasks
	Has difficulty organising tasks and activities	Difficulty organising tasks or activities
	Dislikes or reluctant to engage in tasks requiring sustained mental effort	Avoids, dislikes or reluctant to engage in tasks requiring sustained mental effort
	Is easily distracted by outside stimuli	Loses items required for tasks
	Is often forgetful in daily activities	Easily distracted by extraneous stimuli
	And/or	Forgetful in daily activities
	More than six hyperactive/impulsive symptoms for children up to age 16 and five or more for those over age 17 years	**And**
	Fidgets with hands or feet	Three or more hyperactive/impulsive symptoms, for example
	Cannot remain seated when expected to do so	Fidgets with hands and feet or squirms in seat
	Excessive running about or climbing	Leaves seat in class or where sitting is required
	Has difficulty engaging in quiet activities	Runs or climbs excessively
	Always 'on the go' 'driven by a motor'	Difficulty playing or engaging in leisure activity quietly
	Often talks incessantly	'On the go' or acts as if 'driven by motor'
	Blurts out answers	Talks excessively
	Trouble waiting for their turn	Blurts out answers
	Interrupts or intrudes on others	Difficulty waiting turn
		Interrupts or intrudes on others

common among people with learning disabilities'. The diagnosis is only to be applied where the overall picture meets six criteria:

1 'Symptoms in excess of that which may be expected on the basis of general intelligence, or severity of ID.
2 The age of onset of the disorder should be before 7 years or where historical information is not available "known to be long-standing, extending as far back as available history".
3 The disorder must not be attributable to another psychiatric or physical disorder.
4 There must be a pattern of inattention and distractibility, with poor concentration, flitting and fleeting activity (rather than changing patterns of motor activity), lack of sustained and purposeful actions which must not be attributable to the level of ID.
5 There is an inability to keep still, often noted when affected individuals are seated.
6 The disorder is pervasive and persistent across different situations and over time'.

The clinical presentation of ADHD

While the core features of hyperactivity, impulsivity and inattention can lead to impairment, it is often the associated problems and characteristics that lead the person to seek help from mental health services. Mood instability, irritability and difficult behaviour can cause interpersonal problems and lead to academic under-achievement and difficulty maintaining education or employment opportunities. It can also lead to problems in the community and involvement of the police and criminal justice system. Anxiety and sleep problems frequently co-occur with ADHD. It is known that those with ADHD have a high risk of also having tics, coordination problems and substance misuse (Figure 11.1).

Diagnosis

Clinicians working with people with ID should consider a possible diagnosis of ADHD in those who present with poor attention, impulsive and disorganised behaviours and difficulty sustaining purposeful activity and are hyperactive or restless. The lack of diagnosis for an adult patient previously should not deter a clinician from assessing for the possibility of ADHD as the understanding of assessment and treatment in children with ID continues to lag behind diagnoses of ADHD in generic CAMHS services.

The diagnosis of ADHD requires a detailed developmental and mental assessment and a physical examination to exclude other mental or physical health disorders. It is necessary to exclude psychotic and mood disorders, anxiety disorders, substance misuse, personality disorders and sleep problems.

Detailed information from a family member or carer will be crucial to clarify diagnostic issues, in particular the age of onset of symptoms indicative of ADHD. Both child and adult ADHD scales can be difficult to interpret when there is more

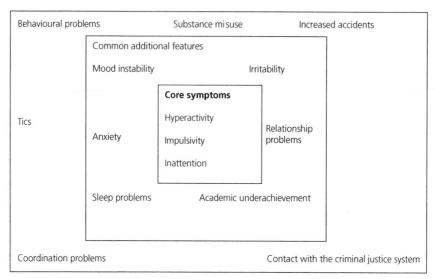

Figure 11.1 Associated conditions and problems.

than a borderline or mild level of ID, and diagnosis based primarily on any ADHD rating scale is not recommended.

The diagnosis of ADHD does require detailed understanding of the ability level of the patient to allow for judgements to be made regarding whether the symptoms are out of context with the ability level. This can be aided by tools such as the Vineland Adaptive Behaviour Scale or the ABAS.

The diagnosis also requires consideration to be given regarding whether the person's environment and care are appropriate to their needs and whether an assessment regarding the functions of their behaviour is required.

Dual diagnosis

Although ICD-10 diagnostic criteria states that ADHD cannot be diagnosed where a pervasive developmental disorder is present, this anomaly has been clarified within the recent NICE guidelines, and ADHD is increasingly being diagnosed in those who have a diagnosis on the autism spectrum. DSM-5 and DC-LD do not have pervasive developmental disorders as exclusion criteria when undertaking a diagnosis of ADHD.

Prevalence

- The prevalence of ADHD is considered to be 5.3% in children and 2.5% in adults without ID.
- The literature and research regarding prevalence of ADHD in those with ID is less clear; however, a recent review indicates increased prevalence of ADHD in

children and adults with ID. It is also suggested that the rate of ADHD increases with the severity of the ID.

- The prevalence of ADHD declines with age in the general adult population. Recent research indicates the possibility of a longer and more persistent course of the disorder in those adults with borderline or mild levels of ID where a more severe presentation and an uneven and less favourable pattern of improvement across the lifespan has been found. The course for those with more severe levels of ID is unclear.

Management

The management of ADHD in children and adults with ID requires a comprehensive plan including psychoeducation, review of their environment, activities, education or employment, assessment and management of their behavioural issues and co-morbidities and consideration given regarding their support needs and those of their family or carers (Algorithm 11.1).

The NICE guideline for children recommends behavioural and parental-based treatment strategies for those under the age of 6 years. Those of school age should be offered a comprehensive package including environmental, behavioural, educational, family and psychological interventions for those with mild or moderate symptoms of ADHD. Where there are severe symptoms of ADHD, or inadequate response to the comprehensive package of care, medication should be offered.

The NICE guidelines recommend adults with ADHD should be offered medication as a first-line treatment unless the person would prefer a psychological approach that could involve a modified form of CBT tailored to the persons' level of ability. It is also recommended that medication should only be commenced by a psychiatrist or non-medical prescriber with training in the diagnosis and management of ADHD. Medication to treat ADHD can be given to those with epilepsy if the seizure activity is stable, liaison with the neurology service, if involved, being considered good practice.

Prior to initiation of medication, a full mental health and social assessment is undertaken, and a full medical history and examination take place. This must include an assessment of exercise syncope, undue breathlessness and other cardiovascular symptoms and note taken of any family history of cardiac disease. There should be examination of the cardiovascular system, and their blood pressure and heart rate should be recorded. An ECG should be requested if there is a past medical or family history of serious cardiac disease, arrhythmia or any abnormality on examination. Height and weight should be recorded as a baseline. There should also be a risk assessment regarding substance misuse or medication diversion.

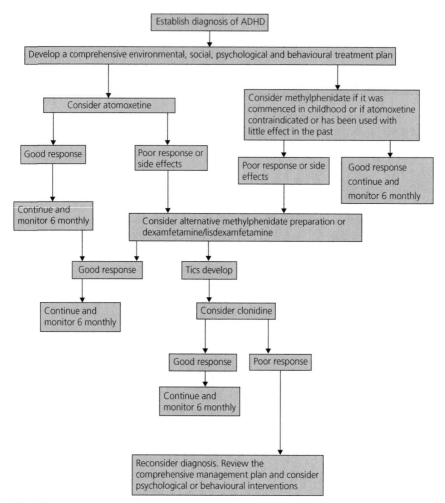

Algorithm 11.1 Management of ADHD in adults with ID.

Role of medication

The medication advised by the NICE guideline includes the CNS stimulants methylphenidate and dexamfetamine and the selective noradrenaline reuptake inhibitor atomoxetine. All three act by increasing the intrasynaptic concentrations of dopamine and noradrenaline in the cortex. It is thought that atomoxetine differs from a stimulant in having less effect on subcortical brain regions associated with motivation and reward.

These medications aim to reduce the core features of ADHD and therefore reduce hyperactivity, impulsivity and inattention in children, adolescents and adults.

The NICE guidelines place methylphenidate as the first-line medication followed by either atomoxetine or dexamfetamine.

It is noted in the guidelines that if treatment with methylphenidate, dexamfetamine and atomoxetine is ineffective, additional medications such as bupropion, clonidine, modafinil and imipramine can be considered by tertiary services. Dopamine antagonists and sedative medications are not recommended for the treatment of ADHD.

Lisdexamfetamine dimesylate was not included in the original NICE guideline, but evidence is included in the NICE Guidance Update 2013. It is a prodrug of dexamfetamine licensed for use in children and young people with ADHD (aged 6 years and above) who have not shown adequate clinical response to methylphenidate. Unlike other medications for ADHD, it is readily soluble and so provides a liquid formulation, which may be of value for children and young people who are unable to swallow tablets or granules.

Atomoxetine has recently been licensed in the UK to be commenced in adults; therefore, as the only licensed preparation for newly diagnosed adults, it would be the preferred medication, unless there are contraindications or if it has been tried and found of little benefit in the past.

Through childhood and adolescence, it is advised to assess the effect of planned and unplanned dose reductions to ensure the core symptoms are still present. This is easier to achieve with the stimulants, as there is an immediate effect compared with atomoxetine where there is a longer effect of treatment and dose changes take up to 6 weeks for maximal effect. It is suggested that dose reductions for young people should be attempted annually, but timing does need to be carefully planned to avoid important events or changes in the person's life. For adults, continuation of ADHD medications are recommended for those who respond well to treatment (Table 11.2).

Monitoring of medication

The NICE guideline recommends the following:
- Use standard symptom and side effect rating scales throughout the course of treatment in additional to clinical reviews.
- For patients receiving methylphenidate, atomoxetine or dexamfetamine, height and weight should be measured at baseline and 3 and 6 months after medication treatment has started and then 6 monthly. These measurements should be plotted on the height weight charts for under 18 year olds. Adults should have their weight and BMI checked s at baseline, 3 months and then 6 monthly to check for weight loss.
- For all medications used to treat ADHD, heart rate and blood pressure should be monitored and recorded on a centile chart before and after each dose change and routinely every 3 months. Those with a sustained resting tachycardia, arrhythmia or systolic blood pressure greater than the 95th percentile (or a

Table 11.2 Choosing a medication for adults.

Medication	Overview of evidence in ADHD
Methylphenidate Usually initiated with low doses of 5 mg upto three times daily. The dose is titrated against symptoms and side effects to maximum of total dose of 100 mg/day. If immediate-release preparation is used, this may be given as divided doses up to four times a day. If extended-release preparations are used, they may be divided into two doses The improvement in symptoms should be seen immediately	The NICE guideline was based upon three placebo-controlled trials in adult populations who did not have ID. There are no randomised placebo-controlled trials for adults with ID and ADHD Clinical evidence for adults with ID has been published using retrospective chart reviews and rating scales indicating that psychostimulants were effective and well tolerated for some of the patients The common side effects include decreased appetite, sleep disturbances, headaches, stomach aches, drowsiness, irritability, tearfulness, increased tics, increased blood pressure and pulse, psychotic symptoms and sensitivity reactions
Dexamfetamine Usually initiated at low dose of 5 mg twice a day. The dose is titrated against symptoms and side effects to maximum of total dose of 60 mg a day in divided doses (usually two to four times a day) The improvement in symptoms should be seen immediately	The NICE guideline was based upon one placebo-controlled study in adults who did not have ID Clinical evidence for adults with ID has been published using retrospective chart reviews and rating scales indicating that psychostimulants were effective and well tolerated for some of the patients Side effects are similar to methylphenidate
Lisdexamfetamine This is prescribed in capsules of 30, 50 or 70 mg. The medication is always initiated at a dose of 30 mg This medication is a prodrug of dexamfetamine and may last for up to 12 hours	The NICE guideline update included evidence using a randomised placebo-controlled trial for use of lisdexamfetamine for children and adolescents. It is noted that it is the only ADHD medication that can be given in liquid formulation. It was not included in the original NICE guideline Side effects are similar to methylphenidate
Atomoxetine For people weighing up to 70 kg/day, the dose should be initiated at 0.5 mg/kg increased after a week to 1.2 mg/kg For those weighing over 70 kg, the initial dose should be 40 mg increased after 7 days to 100 mg usually in divided doses A trial of 6 weeks is required to determine clinical effectiveness	The NICE guideline was based upon three placebo-controlled trials with adults who did not have ID There is no published evidence regarding atomoxetine treatment in adults with ID Atomoxetine is now licensed for the treatment of ADHD in adults

Table 11.2 (*Continued*)

Medication	Overview of evidence in ADHD
	The common side effects include abdominal pain, nausea, vomiting, decreased appetite, weight loss, dizziness, increase in blood pressure and pulse, liver toxicity, seizures, low mood and suicidal behaviours
Clonidine The usual starting dose is 25 μg twice a day increasing after 1–2 weeks to 50 μg twice daily. The maximum dose would be 200 μg twice a day if tolerated	The NICE guideline was based upon one trial with adults without ID who also had a tic disorder
	There are several open-label trials indicating effectiveness of clonidine in children with ADHD and children with autism +/– intellectual disabilities indicating effectiveness Clonidine is not licensed for the treatment of ADHD in children or adults Side effects include hypertensive crisis if withdrawn abruptly, postural hypotension, drowsiness, dry mouth, nausea, vomiting, constipation, headache, depression

Case study 11.1

David is 20 years old and attends college. He has a mild ID and was diagnosed with ADHD when in primary school. David had taken methylphenidate successfully for several years and was receiving 20 mg of the immediate-release preparation three times a day. His mother is concerned because David is refusing to take his methylphenidate and was presenting with high levels of impulsive and aggressive behaviours. His college tutor had spoken to David and his mother stating that his place at the college was at risk due to his behaviour, which was becoming increasingly disruptive for the class.

David was seen by the psychiatrist and a full history and mental state was completed. David denied drinking alcohol or taking any illegal medications. The deterioration coincided with David reducing and stopping the methylphenidate, and there was no evidence of any other mental health concerns. David was able to discuss his distress about being teased at college for taking medication at lunch time. He also said it disrupted his football club as he had to report to the office at a specific time. The psychiatrist was able to discuss alternative slow-release preparations of methylphenidate, lisdexamfetamine or atomoxetine that would continue to provide adequate treatment levels throughout the college day. David chose to restart the slow-release methylphenidate. David was warned that this medication may reduce his lunch time appetite. Side effects were discussed and an information sheet provided so that any side effects could be monitored. He was weighed at the appointment and his blood pressure and pulse was checked. It was agreed that side effects would be discussed in detail at each appointment.

Case study 11.2

> Clare was 19 and had a moderate ID and ADHD. She was diagnosed with ADHD at age 11 and had been taking a slow-release preparation of methylphenidate for several years. The dose had been increased 6 months earlier following deterioration in her behaviour during the transition from home to supported living.
>
> Clare's carers asked for an early review because Clare seemed to be rather low in mood and was losing weight and her sleep had deteriorated.
> - What do you need to consider during the appointment?
> - Could this deterioration be secondary to her methylphenidate treatment?
> - What would be the treatment options at this point?

clinically significant increase) measured on two occasions should have their dose reduced and be referred to a paediatrician or physician.

- During monitoring, it is essential to enquire about appetite loss, sleep disturbance, low mood, anxiety, tics and psychosis and change in seizure frequency as these symptoms can occur at initiation and in longer-term use of the medication and would require dose reduction or discontinuation of the medication.
- Routine blood tests and ECGs are not recommended unless clinically indicated.

Guidelines and practice parameters

National Institute for Health and Care Excellence (NICE). (2009) Attention deficit hyperactivity disorder: diagnosis and management of ADHD in children, young people and adults. NICE clinical guideline 72. London: NICE.

National Institute for Health and Care Excellence (NICE). (2013, July) Attention deficit hyperactivity disorder. Evidence update 45. Manchester: NICE.

Pliszka S; AACAP Work Group on Quality Issues. (2007) Practice parameter for the assessment and treatment of children and adolescents with attention-deficit/hyperactivity disorder. *Journal of the American Academy of Child and Adolescent Psychiatry*. 46(7), 894–921.

Further reading

Coghill D, Banaschewski T, Lecendreux M, et al. (2013) European, randomised, phase 3 study of lisdexamfetamine dimesylate in children and adolescents with attention-deficit/hyperactivity disorder. *European Neuropsychopharmacology*. 23(10), 1208–1218.

Deb S, Dhaliwal A-J, Roy M. (2008) The usefulness of Conners Rating Scales-Revised in screening for attention deficit hyperactivity disorder in children with intellectual disabilities and borderline intelligence. *Journal of Intellectual Disability Research*. 52(part 11), 950–996.

Harfterkamp M, van de Loo-Neus G, Minderaa RB, et al. (2012) A randomized double-blind study of atomoxetine versus placebo for attention-deficit/hyperactivity disorder symptoms in children with autism spectrum disorder. *Journal of the American Academy of Child and Adolescent Psychiatry*. 51(7), 733–741.

McCarthy S, Asherson P, Coghill D, et al. (2009) Attention-deficit hyperactivity disorder: treatment discontinuation in adolescents and young adults. *British Journal of Psychiatry.* 194, 273–277.

Reilly C, Holland N. (2001) Symptoms of attention deficit hyperactivity disorder in children and adults with intellectual disability: a review. *Journal of Applied Research in Intellectual Disabilities.* 24, 291–309.

Seager MC, O'Brien G. (2003) ADHD and learning disability. *Journal of Intellectual Disability Research.* 47(suppl. 1), 26–31.

Simonoff E, Taylor E, Baird G, et al. (2013) Randomized controlled double-blind trial of optimal dose methylphenidate in children and adolescents with severe attention deficit hyperactivity disorder and intellectual disability. *Journal of Child Psychology and Psychiatry.* 54(5), 527–535.

Stores G. (2007) Clinical diagnosis and misdiagnosis of sleep disorders. *Journal of Neurology, Neurosurgery, and Psychiatry.* 78, 1293–1297.

Tan M, Appleton R. (2005) Attention deficit and hyperactivity disorder, methylphenidate, and epilepsy. *Archives of Disease in Childhood.* 90, 57–59.

Xenitidis K, Paliokosta E, Rose E, Maltezos S, Bramham J. (2010) ADHD symptom presentation and trajectory in adults with borderline and mild intellectual disability. *Journal of Intellectual Disability Research.* 54(part 7), 668–677.

CHAPTER 12

Aggressive Behaviour

David Branford[1] & Sabyasachi Bhaumik[2,3]

[1]English Pharmacy Board, Royal Pharmaceutical Society, London, UK
[2]Leicestershire Partnership NHS Trust, Leicester, UK
[3]Department of Health Sciences, University of Leicester, Leicester, UK

> The tendency to aggression is an innate, independent, instinctual disposition in man. It constitutes the powerful obstacle to culture.
>
> *Sigmund Freud*

Definition

Aggression is a severe form of behaviour involving damage to property and/or verbal and/or physical assault to another person. Aggression has been studied extensively by behaviour research scientists, psychologists, psychiatrists and others. Some theories state that aggression is natural, while others suggest that it is acquired as part of social learning. In the context of intellectual disability (ID), frequent or chronic aggression is considered to be a pattern of maladaptive behaviour requiring evaluation and treatment. Aggression that is chronic and persistent poses serious problems for carers and professionals in providing adequate services for people with ID.

Prevalence

People with ID are more susceptible to aggression than the general population. Estimates of prevalence range from 11 to 60% according to the definition of aggression, the sample population and the reliability of the methods of data collection. Although physical and verbal aggression are generally the most frequently reported, many people with ID also engage in other forms of challenging behaviours.

The Frith Prescribing Guidelines for People with Intellectual Disability, Third Edition.
Edited by Sabyasachi Bhaumik, David Branford, Mary Barrett and Satheesh Kumar Gangadharan.
© 2015 John Wiley & Sons, Ltd. Published 2015 by John Wiley & Sons, Ltd.

There are significant gender differences in both the prevalence and type of aggression. Most studies have found that proportionately more males than females engage in aggression, particularly physical aggression, destruction of property, temper tantrums and verbal abuse, although some studies have found no gender difference.

Aggression can be caused by a variety of factors such as difficulties with communication, any physical health problems causing pain or discomfort and mental health problems. In some individuals, aggression can be a learned behaviour from childhood that may have originally served some functions but over the years becomes a pattern of response. In some cases, several of these factors may be contributing to the clinical picture and a thorough assessment is essential prior to intervention commencing. Algorithm 12.1 provides an outline of the assessment process.

Proportionately, more individuals with moderate, severe and profound degrees of ID engage in acts of aggression than those with mild ID. While some studies have shown higher prevalence of aggression in younger age groups, others have found there is no association with age. The prevalence of aggression is higher among people living in long-term institutions (35–38%) than among those in group homes (27%) or community setting (9.7%).

Assessment of the intensity and frequency of the behaviour and risk associated with the behaviour is important in deciding the nature of interventions. An individual with high-risk behaviour or an individual who has the physical ability

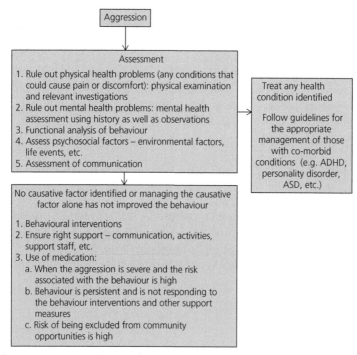

Algorithm 12.1 Assessment of aggression.

Illustrative case study 12.1

Michael, a 24-year-old man with severe intellectual disability and a history of recent increase in aggressive behaviours, is referred to the psychiatrist working in his local intellectual disability service. Michael has been scratching and hitting others. The aggression is most intense in the evening when he returns from the day centre to the residential home that he lives in. While in the past, he would settle down with a drink after returning from the day centre, now he rushes in and out through the back door, hits people on the way and topples furniture. He scratches and hits out a number of staff as well as other residents.

Michael is seen by the psychiatrist, and careful history taking highlights that the behaviour increased following a recent change in his day care. Michael used to attend a traditional day centre where he had the freedom to opt out of activities when he chose to. He would, on those occasions, spend time on his own either in the quiet room or in the sensory garden. His day care is now provided in the community with him accessing various community opportunities. While he used to return home much later than other residents in the past, he now comes back at the same as others to a busy and noisy routine in the home.

The psychiatrist also identified that Michael's father had been hospitalised for some time and has stopped visiting him. He was also noted to be tearful at times, not eating as well as he used to as well as not sleeping well. Observation by nurses trained in behavioural assessment showed that he is not showing much interest in activities, which result in staff returning him often very early in the day.

The psychiatrist initiates an antidepressant that improves Michael's mood, and he becomes more interested in going out. However, the behaviour at the residential home continues. Behavioural assessment identifies that the function of the behaviour is twofold. Firstly, it serves as an escape function at times of overstimulation. Secondly, it serves to gain attention from the staff who were involved in supporting other people. Behaviour improved significantly when a 'quiet area' was introduced to the home, which Michael was able to access on his return from day care, along with extra staff time being allocated to spend on a 1–1 basis with him during the evenings, which included opportunities for visiting his father in the hospital.

and tendency to cause physical injuries would need more active approach including the use of medications to minimise the risk.

Role of medication

The evidence base for medication treatment for aggressive behaviours in isolation remains problematic, as so many trials relate to terms such as problem behaviours or challenging behaviours of which aggressive behaviours may be a component. Also, many medication trials use the Aberrant Behaviour Checklist (ABC) irritability subscale as a proxy for aggressive behaviours. The more recent data is dominated by trials in children. In adults, the NACHBID Health Technology Assessment trial is a most quoted trial.

The NACHBID study by Tyrer and colleagues (2008) conducted a three-arm, parallel-group, randomised trial comparing haloperidol, risperidone and placebo in patients with ID who were showing disruptive behaviour. Despite major methodological problems including under-recruitment and all three arms to the study achieving a parallel drop in the severity of the behaviours within days of the intervention, their conclusion that antipsychotics should no longer be considered an acceptable routine therapy for patients with an ID exhibiting aggressive behaviour flies in the face of much of the rest of the literature. However, as it is the only such trial that meets the NICE criteria in adults, this recommendation has been widely adopted by guidelines. There is a desperate need for further trials to clarify whether this conclusion is valid.

The available data involving controlled trials is summarised in Table 12.1.

Table 12.1 Evidence base for medication treatment of aggressive behaviours in ID.

Medication	Overview of evidence from specific medication trials of benefits in aggressive behaviours
Part 1: Trials in children	
Antipsychotic medications	
Risperidone Usual doses in trials, 1–2 mg daily	Five placebo-controlled studies between 2002 and 2013. Mean ages of participants between ages 7 and 9
	Some evidence of benefit for ABC subscales of irritability, hyperactivity and social withdrawal. These must, however, be considered against adverse effects, most prominently weight gain
	High rate of discontinuation in trials
Aripiprazole Usual doses in trials, 5–10 mg	Two placebo-controlled trial in 2009. Mean ages 9–10 years
	ABC irritability subscale used and diagnosis predominantly autism
	Some evidence of benefit for ABC subscales of irritability. This must, however, be considered against adverse effects, most prominently weight gain. However, this did not seem to cause discontinuation from trials
Part 2a: Trials in adults	
Risperidone	Three placebo-controlled trials since 1998. Only Tyrer et al. (2008) specifically targeted aggression and failed to show any benefits for risperidone over placebo. McDougle (1998) showed greatest benefits but sample predominantly autism
Haloperidol Usual doses, 1–2 mg daily	Licensed for short-term adjunctive management of psychomotor agitation, excitement and violent and dangerous impulsive behaviour
	Haloperidol has been found effective for reducing behavioural symptoms such as hyperactivity, aggression, stereotypies, affective lability and tantrums
	Haloperidol is associated with a high incidence of tardive and withdrawal dyskinesias, and clinical use is significantly limited due to these side effects
Risperidone and haloperidol head to head	No significant difference between groups in terms of improvement, quality of life or adverse events
Quetiapine	A number of very small open trials using low doses have shown limited short-term effects on symptoms such as aggression
Olanzapine	Very limited evidence base. Small trials have shown benefit in alleviating some behavioural symptoms (irritability, hyperactivity/noncompliance and lethargy/withdrawal) associated with autism. Concerns over weight gain and metabolic side effects

Table 12.1 (*Continued*)

Medication	Overview of evidence from specific medication trials of benefits in aggressive behaviours
Olanzapine and risperidone head to head	Amore (2011). Target behaviour predominantly aggression. Although there is some evidence of superiority of risperidone, this did not reach any level of significance
Part 2b: Withdrawal studies in adults	
Zuclopenthixol	Three withdrawal studies (1988, 1992 and 2007). Withdrawal of zuclopenthixol associated with significant increase in aggression and behaviour disorders and reduced adaptive social functioning
General	One discontinuation versus continuation study (Ahmed 2000) showed that 48% of discontinuation group had medication reinstated
Part 3: Other medications	
Lithium	One old study (Craft 1987) showed significant reduction in aggressive behaviours
SSRIs	Four open-label prospective studies using fluoxetine, paroxetine or fluvoxamine lasting 8–16 weeks. Most showed sustained reductions in aggressive behaviours
Valproate	One open-label studies and two in children with inconclusive results

Discussion case study 12.2

Amy, a 48-year-old woman with moderate intellectual disability (ID), is admitted to the local inpatient unit following a number of assaults on staff as well as other people with ID. She lives with her elderly mother and attends the day centre. The behaviour was first reported by the day centre; however, on further clarification, her mother revealed that the behaviour has been ongoing since Amy's dad died 18 months ago, and the mother has many bruises on her arms. She, however, stated that her daughter never means to hurt her but that Amy has been getting 'very difficult' about her personal care.

On admission, Amy is found to be in a poorly kempt state. She refuses to be separated from a bag of torn up papers, which she brought in to the hospital with her, and spends hours rearranging the papers in piles. Her communication consists mainly of repetitive phrases. She tends to sit alone and is clearly aversive to physical touch and loud noises.

1 What assessments would she need?
2 What the diagnostic possibilities?
3 What treatment options would you consider?
4 Is there a role for medication here?

When choosing a medication, it is vital to be clear what symptom(s) to target. The individual with ID and carers should be involved in the decision-making process, with the individual giving informed consent if they have the capacity to do so. For individuals lacking capacity, best interest principles should be followed. In all cases, the prescriber should have a clear plan for the review of progress and termination of treatment where the treatment is not working or no more required.

Guidelines

Deb S, Clarke D, Unwin G. (2006, September) Using medications to manage behavioural prob-lems among adults with a learning disability. DATABID. www.LD-Medication.bham.ac.uk (accessed 8 January 2015).

National Institute for Health and Care Excellence. (2005) Violence: the short-term management of disturbed/violent behaviour in in-patient psychiatric settings and emergency departments. http://www.nice.org.uk/nicemedia/pdf/cg025fullguideline.pdf (accessed 8 January 2015).

References

Amore M, Bertelli M, Villani D, Tamborini S, Rossi M. (2011) Olanzapine vs. risperidone in treating aggressive behaviours in adults with intellectual disability: a single blind study. *J Intellect Disabil Res* 55(2): 210–218.

Ahmed Z, Fraser W, Kerr MP, et al. (2000) Reducing antipsychotic medication in people with a learning disability. *Br J Psych* 176:42–46.

Craft M, Ismail IA, Krishnamurti D, et al. (1987) Lithium in the treatment of aggression in mentally handicapped patients: a double-blind trial. *Br J Psych* 150:685–689.

McDougle CJ, Holmes JP, Carlson DC, Pelton GH, Cohen DJ, Price LH. (1998) A double-blind, placebo-controlled study of risperidone in adults with autistic disorder and other pervasive developmental disorders. *Arch Gen Psych* 55:633–641.

Tyrer P, Oliver-Africano PC, Ahmed Z, et al. (2008) Risperidone, haloperidol, and placebo in the treatment of aggressive challenging behaviour in patients with intellectual disability: a randomised controlled trial. *Lancet* 371:57–63.

Further reading

Benson BA, Brooks WT. (2008) Aggressive challenging behaviour and intellectual disability. *Current Opinion in Psychiatry* 21(5):454–458.

Brylewski J, Duggan L. (2007) Antipsychotic medication for challenging behavior in people with intellectual disability: a systematic review of randomized controlled trials. *Cochrane Database of Systematic Reviews* (3):CD000377.

Davies L, Oliver C. (2013) Age related prevalence of aggression and self-injury in persons with an intellectual disability. *Research in Developmental Disabilities* 34:764–775.

Deb S, Sohanpal SK, Soni R, Unwin G, Lenôtre L. (2007) The effectiveness of antipsychotic medication in the management of behaviour problems in adults with intellectual disabilities. *Journal of Intellectual Disability Research* 51(10):766–777.

Deb S, Unwin G, Deb T. (2014) Characteristics and the trajectory of psychotropic medication use in general and antipsychotics in particular among adults with an intellectual disability who exhibit aggressive behaviour. *Journal of Intellectual Disability Research* 59:11–25. doi: 10.1111/jir.12119.

Matson JL, Wilkins J. (2008) Antipsychotic medications for aggression in intellectual disability. *Lancet* 371:9–10.

Roy D, Hoffman P, Dudas M, Mendelowitz A. (2013) Pharmacologic management of aggression in adults with intellectual disability. *Journal of Intellectual Disability – Diagnosis and Treatment* 1:28–43.

Tsiouris JA. (2010) Pharmacotherapy for aggressive behaviours in persons with intellectual disabilities: treatment or mistreatment? *Journal of Intellectual Disability Research* 54(1):1–16.

CHAPTER 13

Self-Injurious Behaviour

Asit Biswas[1] & Sabyasachi Bhaumik[1,2]

[1]Leicestershire Partnership NHS Trust, Leicester, UK
[2]Department of Health Sciences, University of Leicester, Leicester, UK

> Self-injury can be one of the most distressing and difficult behaviours that parents, carers, family members and people themselves may be faced with.
>
> *National Autistic Society*

Definition

Self-injurious behaviour (SIB) may be defined as non-accidental self-inflicted acts causing damage to, or destruction of, body tissue and carried out without suicidal ideation or intent.

Clinical presentation

SIB may be viewed as a symptom of a psychiatric disorder, or in the context of behaviour arising from maladaptive learning, or in association with behavioural phenotypes. SIB may present as head banging, head hitting or face slapping, self-biting to the hands or other parts of the body, removing scabs from old wounds, self-pinching or scratching, hair pulling and eye poking. It often presents in multiple forms in the same person.

SIB can be symptomatic of many underlying causes, including communication difficulties, physical health problems and pain. Clinically significant SIB presents serious challenges to professionals and may cause severe distress to carers. SIB

Table 13.1 Clinical SIB subtypes.

Subtype	Central feature	Neurotransmitter system
Extreme self-inflicted tissue damage	Insensitivity to pain	Opiate
Repetitive and stereotypic	Features of autism	Dopamine
Agitation when SIB is interrupted	Obsessive–compulsive behaviour	Serotonin
Heightened anxiety	High arousal (agitation and SIB co-occur)	Noradrenaline
Mixed	Two or more of above subtype	Multiple

Source: Adapted from Mace and Mauck (1995). © Wiley.

may also reduce an individual's quality of life, for example, by exclusion from community-based educational facilities or day services.

Using a biomedical model, clinical subtypes are determined by the presence of certain clinical features (Table 13.1, adapted from Mace and Mauck's model).

Prevalence

The point prevalence of SIB differs between studies, depending on the definition of SIB, the methodology used and the population studied. A prevalence of 1.7–41% has been reported in adults with intellectual disability (ID), with 4.2–16% in community-based studies. In large-scale population-based community survey, SIB with sufficient severity to cause tissue damage was noted in 5% of adults.

The prevalence of SIB shows a curvilinear relationship with age, being more common in adolescents and young adults than in children or older people. There is no significant gender difference in the overall prevalence of SIB. The frequency of SIB increases with the severity of ID. SIB has also been reported more frequently in people who are blind or have speech problems or autism. SIB is associated with Lesch–Nyhan syndrome, fragile X syndrome, Cornelia de Lange syndrome, Prader–Willi syndrome, Rett syndrome and Smith–Magenis syndrome.

Assessment and management

Assessment
Assessment should take account of all the aetiological features outlined earlier unless an obvious remediable cause explains the behaviour. Assessment should be multidisciplinary since a combination of approaches is more likely to succeed than a single one (Algorithm 13.1).

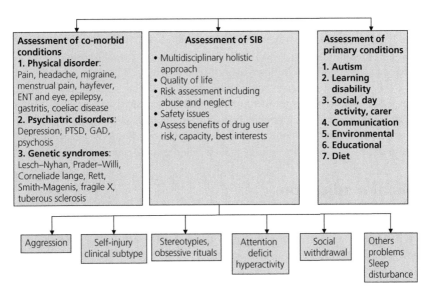

Algorithm 13.1 Assessment of SIB.

Illustrative case study 13.1

Sam is a 29-year-old male with severe ID, epilepsy and autism. He has long-standing SIB in the form of head banging, self-biting and scratching. Sam is re-referred urgently to the ID psychiatrist with 'mood swings' and escalating self-biting. History taking reveals an alternating pattern of 3 days of arousal/insomnia/increased SIB, followed by a week of quietness/social withdrawal/variable appetite. There is no contributory physical or environmental cause.

The psychiatrist suspects a rapid-cycling mood disorder and prescribes a mood stabiliser with benefit to his mood fluctuations. Review several months later reveals an improvement in self-biting; however, head banging continues to be a concern. Observations carried out at the day centre by a member of the ID nursing team reveal that Sam's head banging is associated with high physical anxiety levels. Behavioural strategies to reduce his anxieties including relaxation and trampolining are tried with limited success; a trial of propranolol is given, with significant improvement, and this allows Sam to successfully engage with the behavioural strategies, which further reduces his arousal levels.

Behavioural programmes

In view of the possibility of serious medication side effects, a behaviour programme should be tried first. A behavioural monitoring programme should remain in place during treatment with psychotropic medication. This should include systematic direct observations and, in special cases, the use of rating scales such as the Aberrant Behaviour Checklist or Self-Injury Trauma Scale.

Medication should only be used after behavioural methods and other approaches have been tried. The treatment of choice depends on the subtype of SIB (see Table 13.3). Some people who display predominantly pain insensitivity benefit from opiate antagonists. Low doses of antipsychotics may be useful for autistic individuals displaying stereotypies and challenging SIB. Where a compulsive element is suspected, selective serotonin reuptake inhibitors (SSRIs) or a tricyclic antidepressant such as clomipramine may be useful. Individuals with high levels of anxiety or arousal often respond to mood-stabilising medications or propranolol. Certain syndromal associations may need a different approach to manage SIB.

Role of medication

There is evidence from both human and animal research for a role for dysregulation of biological systems in SIB and evidence for the efficacy of corresponding pharmacological interventions in some cases.

Biological model

The biological model in SIB is based on three types of neurotransmitters: dopamine, opioids and serotonin.

Dopamine

Responses to dopamine agonists such as pemoline and findings in Lesch–Nyhan syndrome lend support to the dopamine receptor oversensitivity theory. D_1 receptors are thought to be the principal dopamine receptors involved, a concept with therapeutic implications since many traditional antipsychotics have little effect at these sites. Antipsychotics such as olanzapine and clozapine are more active at these receptors and have been successful in treating SIB.

Opioids

Studies showing raised plasma beta-endorphin levels in people with SIB or a reduction in SIB in response to administration of opiate-blocking agents support the involvement of endogenous opiates. However, it is unclear whether SIB is the cause or an effect of raised endogenous opiates.

Serotonin

Low levels of serotonin have been found in people with Cornelia de Lange syndrome and SIB. Case reports suggest a treatment response to SSRIs such as fluoxetine and tricyclic antidepressants such as clomipramine.

Choosing a medication

The evidence base for medication treatment in SIB remains limited; however, the available data is summarised in Table 13.2.

Table 13.2 Evidence base for medication treatment in self-injurious behaviour in people with intellectual disability.

Medication	Overview of evidence from specific medication trials of benefits in self-injurious behaviour
Antipsychotics	
Risperidone	The best available evidence is for risperidone
Usual doses, 1–2 mg daily	In a double-blind crossover trial of risperidone (Zarcone et al., 2001) described a positive effect using the Aberrant Behaviour Checklist as an outcome variable. A positive effect for 50% of the sample was reported, as evidenced by a 50% reduction in scores on the Aberrant Behaviour Checklist. Risperidone is effective for short-term treatment of aggression, temper outbursts and self-injurious behaviour (SIB)
	No significant change in SIB was noted by using doses of 0.02–0.06 mg/kg/day versus placebo in a 6-week double-blind parallel-group study in 115 children
Aripiprazole	No randomised controlled trials. Two open-label studies – small numbers – 92–100% response rate
Olanzapine	Limited evidence base. Hollander et al. (2006) found global improvement using doses of 10 mg/day versus placebo in 11 concerns over sedation, weight gain and metabolic side effects
Ziprasidone	No randomised controlled trials. Two open-label studies with small numbers. A 50–70% response rate was noted
Quetiapine	No randomised controlled trials. Four open-label studies with small numbers. A response rate between 22 and 60% was reported
Antidepressants	
SSRIs	In a single-case study, an open trial of sertraline using a baseline intervention single-case experimental design demonstrated a decrease in SIB when the medication was used in combination with a behavioural intervention (Mace et al., 2001)
Clomipramine	Comparison of clomipramine versus placebo found no statistically significant benefit for any outcome measure, which included SIB rate and intensity, stereotypy and adverse events. However, it showed clinically significant improvement in the rate and intensity of SIB and stereotypy
Opiate antagonists	
Naltrexone	One of the naltrexone versus placebo trials reported that naltrexone had clinically significant effects ($\geq$33% reduction) on the daily rates of three of the four participants' most severe form of SIB and modest to substantial reductions in SIB for all participants; however, this study did not report on statistical significance. Another trial reported that naltrexone attenuated SIB in all four participants, with 25 and 50 mg doses producing a statistically significant decrease in SIB (P value <0.05). Another trial (eight people) indicated that naltrexone administration was associated with significantly fewer days of high frequency self-injury and significantly more days with low-frequency self-injury. Naltrexone had different effects depending on the form and location of self-injury. Another trial with only 26 participants found that neither single-dose (100 mg) nor long-term (50 and 150 mg) naltrexone treatment had any therapeutic effect on SIB

Table 13.3 Rationale of drug selection based on clinical sub-type.

Subtype	Clinical features	Psychotropic medications (aim for monotherapy if possible)
Extreme self-inflicted tissue damage (Opiate)	*History of severe SIB* Fractures, extensive scarring, lacerations >3 × 3 cm², cauliflower ear, auto-amputation, loss of consciousness Signs of little distress when inflicting self-injury – crying, screaming Targeting the head/face/hands/fingers	Opiate antagonists Naltrexone

Repetitive and stereotypic (Dopamine)	*History of repetitive and stereotypic SIB*
	 Topography of actions are similar, not variable, for example, hand mouthing, repeated rubbing
	 Short duration between repetitive action (1–10 seconds)
	 Tissue damage occurs due to repetitive injury
	 Other non-SIB stereotypic behaviours are also present
		Antipsychotics (small doses)
		 Atypicals:
		   Risperidone
		   Amisulpride
		   Quetiapine
		   Olanzapine
		 Older medications:
		   Haloperidol
		   Levomepromazine
		   Chlorpromazine

Agitation when SIB is interrupted (Serotonin)	Obsessive–compulsive behaviour Agitation or distress when SIB is interrupted, for example, crying, hyperventilation, aggression, pacing Mean rate of SIB is usually >100 incidents per hour SIB stops during another activity but resumes within 30 seconds of its completion	Selective serotonin reuptake inhibitors (SSRIs) Fluoxetine TCAs (tricyclics) Clomipramine
Heightened anxiety (Noradrenaline)	High arousal – tachycardia, raised BP, pacing, agitation, screaming SIB rates vary considerably (>50%) between sessions and settings Topographies consist of hitting self, head banging Sleep and/or appetite disturbance Slowing of processing of information presented Anxious affect Preoccupied in deep thoughts	*Anxiolytics* Propranolol Pregabalin *TCAs* Amitriptyline (low dose) *Mood stabilisers* Lithium carbonate Carbamazepine Sodium valproate
Mixed (Multiple)	A combination of features in two or more of the subtypes described before Most common presentation	One or more medication classes depending on predominant subtype

Discussion case study 13.2

Lisa is a 21-year-old Caucasian female with mild ID. She moved into residential care four years ago, after her parents had difficulties managing her behaviours. She currently is unable to access day activities outside the home due to challenging behaviour. Behaviours include aggression (biting others, hitting out at others, screaming, shouting) and SIB (slapping face, head banging, biting wrists).

Staff report Lisa to be experiencing marked mood fluctuations and a disturbed sleep pattern. They have also noticed that Lisa's SIB increases after family visits and premenstrually. Lisa's placement is now at risk.

- What are the diagnostic possibilities?
- What treatment strategies could be tried?
- What would be your first choice of medication and why?

A Cochrane review (2013) found weak evidence in included trials that any active medication was more effective than placebo for people with ID demonstrating SIB. Due to sparse data, an absence of power and statistical significance, and high risk of bias for four of the included trials, they were unable to reach any definite conclusions about the relative benefits of naltrexone or clomipramine compared to placebo.

When choosing a medication, it is vital to be clear what symptom(s) you are targeting. Table 13.3 summarises the key subtype of SIB that needs targeting for optimum treatment.

References

Hollander E, Wasserman S, Swanson EN, et al. (2006). A double-blind placebo-controlled pilot study of olanzapine in childhood/adolescent pervasive developmental disorder. *Journal of Child and Adolescent Psychopharmacology*, 16(5), 541–548.

Mace FC, Mauck JE (1995). Biobehavioural diagnosis and treatment of self-injury. *Mental Retardation and Developmental Disabilities Research Reviews*, 1, 104–110.

Mace FC, Blum NJ, Sierp BJ, et al. (2001). Differential response of operant self-injury to pharmacologic versus behavioural treatment. *Journal of Developmental and Behavioral Pediatrics*, 22, 85–91.

Rana F, Gormez A, Varghese S (2013). Drugs as treatment for self-injurious behaviour in adults with intellectual disabilities. www.cochrane.org/CD009084/BEHAV_drugs-as-treatment-for-self-injurious-behaviour-in-adults-with-intellectual-disabilities (accessed 3 March 2015).

Zarcone JR, Hellings JA, Crandall K, et al. (2001). Effects of Risperidone on aberrant behavior of persons with developmental disabilities: a double-blind crossover. *American Journal of Mental Retardation*, 106, 525–538.

Further reading

Aman MG (1993). Efficacy of psychotropic medications for reducing self-injurious behaviour in the developmental disabilities. *Annals of Clinical Psychiatry*, 5, 177–188.

Casner JA, Weinheimer B, Gualtieri CT (1996). Naltrexone and self-injurious behaviour: a retrospective population study. *Journal of Clinical Psychopharmacology*, 16, 389–394.

Cooper SA, Smiley E, Allan LM, et al. (2009). Adults with intellectual disabilities: prevalence, incidence and remission of self-injurious behaviour and related factors. *Journal of Intellectual Disability Research*, 53, 200–216.

Furniss F, Biswas AB (2012). Recent research on aetiology, development and phenomenology of self-injurious behaviour in people with intellectual disabilities: a systematic review and implications for treatment. *Journal of Intellectual Disability Research*, 56(5), 453–475.

Lewis MH, Bodfish JW, Powell SB, Parker DE, Golden RN (1996). Clomipramine treatment for self-injurious behaviour of individuals with mental retardation: a double-blind comparison with placebo. *American Journal of Mental Retardation*, 100, 654–665.

McDonough M, Hillery J, Kennedy N (2000). Olanzapine for chronic, stereotypic self-injurious behaviour: a pilot study in seven adults with intellectual disability. *Journal of Intellectual Disability Research*, 44, 677–684.

Ricketts RW, Goza AB, Ellis CR, Singh YN, Singh NN, Cooke JC 3rd (1993). Fluoxetine treatment of severe self-injury in young adults with mental retardation. *Journal of the American Academy of Child & Adolescent Psychiatry*, 32, 865–869.

Ruedrich S, Swales TP, Fossaceca C, Toliver J, Rutkowski A (1999). Effect of divalproex sodium on aggression and self-injurious behaviour in adults with intellectual disability: a retrospective review. *Journal of Intellectual Disability Research*, 43, 105–111.

Schroeder SR (1996). Dopaminergic mechanisms in self-injury. *Psychology in Mental Retardation and Developmental Disabilities*, 22, 10–13.

CHAPTER 14

Anxiety Disorders

Avinash Hiremath[1], Sabyasachi Bhaumik[1,2] & Khalid Nawab[3]

[1]Leicestershire Partnership NHS Trust, Leicester, UK
[2]Department of Health Sciences, University of Leicester, Leicester, UK
[3]NHS Lanarkshire, Glasgow, UK

> Even if she be not harmed, her heart may fail her in so much and so many horrors; and hereafter she may suffer – both in waking, from her nerves, and in sleep, from her dreams.
>
> *Bram Stoker,* Dracula

Definition

Anxiety is a universal experience. It is characterised by distinct physiological and psychological symptoms, which when present at a frequency and/or severity that causes subjective distress present as a disorder. As a mental disorder, it ranks as one of the most common to afflict the population. There are several types of anxiety disorders including phobias (agoraphobia, social phobia and specific phobias), panic disorder, generalised anxiety disorder and obsessive–compulsive disorder.

Clinical presentation

The symptoms of anxiety, including diagnostic criteria for specific anxiety disorders, are well described in all diagnostic classifications (ICD-10, DSM-5 and DC-LD). As with other mental disorders, there is a reliance on understanding the subjective experience, which requires the cognitive ability to understand and appraise the experience and the linguistic skills to articulate it. Diagnosing these disorders in people with intellectual disabilities (ID), a large proportion of who have significant communication difficulties, can present a significant challenge.

The Frith Prescribing Guidelines for People with Intellectual Disability, Third Edition.
Edited by Sabyasachi Bhaumik, David Branford, Mary Barrett and Satheesh Kumar Gangadharan.
© 2015 John Wiley & Sons, Ltd. Published 2015 by John Wiley & Sons, Ltd.

When considering a diagnosis of anxiety disorder in a person with ID, the following factors need to be borne in mind:
- Mental disorders, especially anxiety disorders, can be overlooked in people with ID due to diagnostic overshadowing.
- Where patients struggle to articulate their experience verbally or with communication aids, attention needs to be paid to the behavioural correlates of specific symptoms of anxiety (Box 14.1) to support a diagnostic assessment.
- Due rigour must be exercised with some symptoms that may be challenging to define phenomenologically or may be present in other developmental disorders (Box 14.2).

Due to the above, a diligent approach must be adopted when assessing a patient for symptoms of anxiety. This includes:
- Sufficient time to interview the patient and the carers, adopting a communication approach based on patient needs.
- Sufficient time to observe patient in various settings.
- Rule out medical disorders and medical treatments that may present with symptoms of anxiety disorders.
- When considering a differential diagnosis with other developmental disorders, a detailed history may establish symptoms as either developmental or new onset.
- Consider the use of validated tools (PAS-ADD).

Box 14.1 Examples of behavioural correlates of anxiety symptoms

1. Dry mouth	Drinking excessive fluids
2. Sensation of shortness of breath	Hyperventilation
3. Anxiety	Increased arousal (sweating, clammy extremities, tachycardia) avoidance, self-injurious behaviour
4. Panic	Tremors, agitation, increased motor activity

Box 14.2 Examples of symptoms causing diagnostic confusion

1. Repetitive behaviours: present in both OCD and autism
2. Social avoidance: can be a feature of intellectual disability, autism and/or social phobia
3. Specific phobias: may be appropriate to the mental age of the patient, in terms of cognitive development
4. Symptoms of anxiety may be a behavioural phenotype in some syndromes, for example, social anxiety in fragile X syndrome

Prevalence

Depending on the criteria used for diagnosis, the prevalence of anxiety disorders in people with ID ranges from 2.4 to 3.8%. The prevalence rates for specific disorders were generalised anxiety disorder 1.7%, agoraphobia 0.7%, social phobia 0.3%, panic disorder 0.2% and post-traumatic stress disorder 0.3%. Some of the variables associated with anxiety disorders (and other mental disorders) include severe to profound ID, female sex, high number of life events in the preceding 12-month period and higher number of primary care consultations in the preceding 12-month period.

Management

Psychological treatment

Patients with ID, especially those with moderate to severe ID, who are suffering from anxiety disorders are likely to under-report their experience and present with behavioural agitation rather than cognitive symptoms. Much of the evidence in ID, therefore, is based on behavioural treatments focussed on relaxation training. The evidence for cognitive behaviour therapy is based on specific symptom areas like anger, fire-setting, etc., and it is difficult to hypothesise whether these treatments would therefore work in anxiety disorders.

For people with mild ID, the results from mainstream research can be generalised and a person-centred cognitive behavioural approach with appropriate reasonable adjustments should be considered. For those with moderate to severe ID, however, the evidence base – and therefore the utility of behaviour or cognitive behaviour therapy – is questionable.

Medication

As with non-drug treatments, there is a dearth of good quality research into the use of various medications in the anxiety disorders in people with ID. Most of the literature is based on the use of SSRIs in challenging behaviour, some of which have been considered as a result of anxiety disorders. There are no randomised controlled trials for any of the SSRIs or other medications for the treatment of anxiety disorders in people with ID. The support for using medications is therefore based on the research into these medications and the good practice guidance generated for the mainstream population and clinical consensus publications.

When using medications, especially SSRIs, attention must be given to both the initiation and discontinuation phases, which are likely to cause some anxiety and distress. The following principles may be considered:

1 The use of benzodiazepines for a few days when commencing an SSRI may help attenuate this distress.

2 When stopping medications, it is advisable to taper these slower than in mainstream population as the experience of discontinuation symptoms may, in itself, present as severe anxiety.

3 In physically healthy individuals, the mean therapeutic dose must always be considered for symptom remission and maintenance. There is no evidence to suggest that people with ID who are in good health may not be able to tolerate the maximum licensed dose of these medications.

4 Most of the medications used to treat anxiety tend to influence the seizure threshold. It is therefore advised to exercise caution with dose escalation.

5 Some of the SSRIs are associated with gastrointestinal side effects that are relatively less tolerated by people with ID. As this may present with distress, which may not be distinguishable from the experience of anxiety, it may be worthwhile starting with much lower doses retrying these medications rather than concluding it as a failed therapeutic trial (Algorithms 14.1, 14.2 and 14.3).

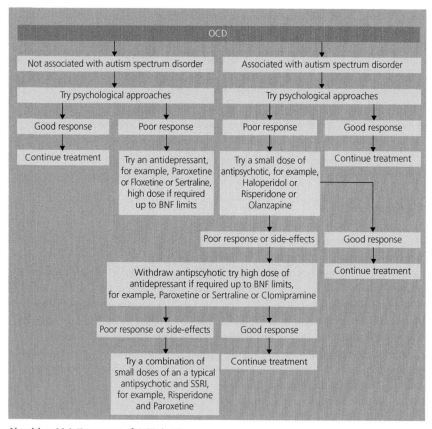

Algorithm 14.1 Treatment of OCD in ID.

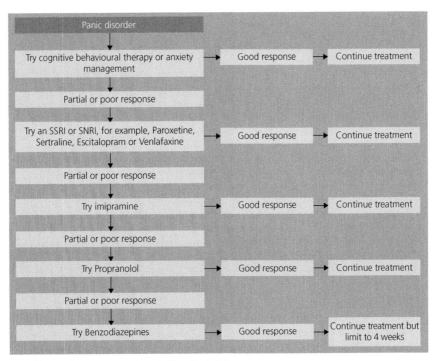

Algorithm 14.2 Treatment of panic disorder in ID.

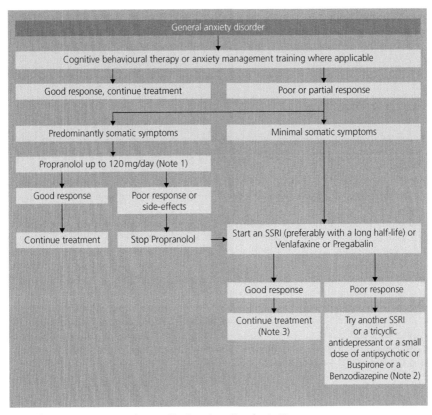

Algorithm 14.3 Treatment of generalised anxiety disorder in ID.

Illustrative case study 14.1

> Patrick, a 25-year-old man with mild ID, presented with agitation, ritualistic behaviour and disengagement from his usual planned activities. His carers reported he was spending a lot of time in the bathrooms and wandering into other service users' rooms to check their light switches and was slapping his head while muttering about 'bad thoughts'.
>
> A detailed assessment excluded environmental changes, physical health problems and other developmental disorders including autism. Mental state examination revealed obsessive fears, obsessive doubts and compulsive rituals. An initial treatment plan based on CBT was advised. However, Patrick's anxiety and behavioural disruption necessitated the consideration of medications to reduce the anxiety, improve social functioning and preserve the care structure, in light of potential retaliation from other service users.
>
> An SSRI was prescribed, with cautious escalation of the dose within the recommended range, resulting in reduction of symptoms and improved functioning. Patrick was then able to engage with CBT and his placement was successfully maintained.

Discussion case study 14.2

> Margaret, a 32-year-old woman with moderate to severe ID, living with her family, presented to services with a recent increase in agitation and self-injurious behaviours. Due to the level of irritability and agitation, she had been excluded from attending day centre activities. She was also reporting headaches and backache. Carers reported she was continuing to be unusually restless and was unable to focus on activities.
> - What is your differential diagnosis?
> - What investigations are indicated?
> - What support could Margaret be given to help her communicate her symptoms?
> - What is the role of medication if Margaret is experiencing anxiety symptoms?

Further reading

Aman MG, Arnold LE, Armstrong SC. (1999) Review of serotonergic agents and perseverative behavior in patients with developmental disabilities. *Ment Retard Dev Disabil Res Rev* 5(4):279–289.

Antochi R, Stavrakaki C, Emery PC. (2003) Psychopharmacological treatments in persons with dual diagnosis of psychiatric disorders and developmental disabilities. *Postgrad Med J* 79:139–146.

Bodfish JW, Madison JT. (1993) Diagnosis and fluoxetine treatment of compulsive behavior disorder of adults with mental retard. *Am J Ment Retard* 98:360–367.

Cooray SE, Bakala A. (2005) Anxiety disorders in people with learning disabilities. *Adv Psychiatr Treat* 11:355–361.

Masi G, Luccherino L. (1997) Psychiatric illness in mental retardation: an update on pharmacotherapy. *Panminerva Med* 39(4):299–304.

National Institute for Health and Care Excellence. (2011, January) Generalised anxiety disorder and panic disorder (with or without agoraphobia) in adults: management in primary, secondary and community care. NICE guidance CG 113. http://publications.nice.org.uk/generalised-anxiety-disorder-and-panic-disorder-with-or-without-agoraphobia-in-adults-cg113 (accessed 8 January 2015).

Pruijssers AC, Van Meijel B, Maaskant M, Nijssen W, van Achterberg T. (2014) The relationship between challenging behaviour and anxiety in adults with intellectual disabilities: a literature review. *J Intellect Disabil Res* 58(2):162–171. Special Issue: Mental Health and Intellectual Disability: XXIXIII.

Wiener K, Lamberti JS. (1993) Sertraline and mental retardation with obsessive-compulsive disorder [letter]. *Am J Psychiatry* 150:1270.

Werry JS. (1998) Anxiolytics and sedatives. In: Reiss S, Aman MG, eds. *Psychotropic medications and developmental disabilities. The international consensus handbook.* Columbus, OH: Ohio State University Nisonger Center; 201–214.

CHAPTER 15

Depression

Avinash Hiremath, Shweta Gangavati, Rohit Gumber & Mary Barrett
Leicestershire Partnership NHS Trust, Leicester, UK

> But with the slow menace of a glacier, depression came on. No one had any measure of
> its progress; no one had any plan for stopping it. Everyone tried to get out of its way.
> *Frances Perkins (American Politician 1882–1965)*

Definition

Depression refers to a wide range of mental health problems characterised by the absence of a positive affect (a loss of interest and enjoyment in ordinary things and experiences), low mood and a range of associated emotional, cognitive, physical and behavioural symptoms.

Distinguishing the mood clinically changes between significant degrees of depression (e.g. major depression) and those occurring 'normally' remains problematic, and it is best to consider the symptoms of depression as occurring on a continuum of severity (Lewinsohn et al., 2000).

The identification of major depression is based not only on its severity but also on persistence, the presence of other symptoms and the degree of functional and social impairment. However, there appears to be no hard-and-fast 'cut-off' between 'clinically significant' and 'normal' degrees of depression; the greater the severity of depression, the greater the morbidity and adverse consequences (Lewinsohn et al., 2000; Kessing, 2007).

The Frith Prescribing Guidelines for People with Intellectual Disability, Third Edition.
Edited by Sabyasachi Bhaumik, David Branford, Mary Barrett and Satheesh Kumar Gangadharan.
© 2015 John Wiley & Sons, Ltd. Published 2015 by John Wiley & Sons, Ltd.

Prevalence

There is a general lack of suitable diagnostic criteria, which adds to the difficulty of accurately delineating the size of the problem; however, studies suggest that affective disorders, particularly depression, are often underdiagnosed and inadequately treated in people with intellectual disability (ID). Studies of the point prevalence of depression in adults with ID show levels between 1.3 and 3.7%. Older people with ID may be more prone to depression, with 8.9% of hospital residents and 6.7% of community residents affected.

Clinical presentation

People with depression and mild ID may present in a similar fashion to the general population and be able to articulate their emotional state; however, for those individuals with moderate or more severe ID, the clinician will often be reliant on observable features such as a change in sleep pattern, loss of appetite, reduced interest in activities, agitation, aggression and self-injury. The presentation may be atypical due to the presence of associated conditions such as autism spectrum disorders (ASD) (see following text) or modified by other medication the person is taking, for example, mood stabilisers/antiepileptic or antipsychotic drugs.

Key factors to consider are the following:
- The onset of depression tends to be more insidious and the changes less dramatic than general population.
- Presenting features may be regression/loss of adaptive skills, withdrawal from normal activities, aggression and self-injury.
- The symptoms of depression may be misattributed to the ID itself.
- Observable signs and symptoms may be modified by medication, for example, early morning wakening may be masked by the sedative effect of an antipsychotic being prescribed for challenging behaviour.
- Anxiety, a frequent co-morbid symptom, may be expressed in the form of avoidance behaviour or autonomic features, which are situation specific.
- Due to limited verbal skills/insight into the internal emotional state by the person with ID, the clinician may have to rely more on observable signs than on self-report.
- Influence of environment: poor physical/social circumstances can have a significant impact, especially if the person with ID has little control/influence over their living circumstances.

Clinical presentation of depression in ID.

Core symptoms	• Tearfulness
	• Social withdrawal
	• Low mood
	• Irritability
	• Reduced energy
	• Fatigue
	• Increased/decreased appetite with increased/decreased weight
	• Insomnia/hypersomnia
Behavioural symptoms	• Aggression
	• Self-injurious behaviour
	• Screaming
	• Temper tantrums
	• Incontinence
Other symptoms	• Hypochondriacal symptoms: headache, abdominal pain, vomiting
	• Generalised deterioration in social relationships and self-care skills
	• Erotomanic delusions (rare)
	• Pica (rare)

Depression and Down syndrome

A review of the literature by Walker et al. (2011) stated that there is no real evidence of increased prevalence of depression in people with Down syndrome compared to other causes of ID.

Depression in people with ASD

Kannabiran and McCarthy (2009) reported that in people with ASD, the onset of or an increase in maladaptive behaviours such as repeating, hoarding, touching and tapping behaviours may be the presenting features in depression.

Depression in people with ID and epilepsy

According to Turky et al. (2008), they have found that there is an increased risk of unspecified disorders, depression and dementia in adults with ID and epilepsy.

Dementia

Symptoms of depression may commonly present in a person who is experiencing the onset of dementia. The treatment of the depression may result in a certain degree of improvement, for example, lifting of mood; however, the underlying dementia will remain and needs to be assessed and treated accordingly.

Schizophrenia

Following successful treatment of a psychotic illness with antipsychotic medication, symptoms of depression may then emerge. This is referred to as revealed depression.

Life events

Life events that result in a loss for the person with ID may trigger depression. Life events in the ID population may vary from those typically seen in the general population. Changes such as a sudden loss of key worker or change of day-care facility/peer group need to be considered.

Bereavement for an individual with ID may be a particularly threatening life event, especially if it results in rapid changes in personal circumstances. Intense reactions such as self-injury may be observed in as many as 10–15% of reactions to grief, and depressive symptoms are frequent.

Suicide

Although suicide is rarely reported in people with ID, suicidal behaviours including threats of suicide and self-injurious behaviour with suicidal intent have been described. One study found that suicidal individuals tend to be young and to have borderline ID and chronic poor health or physical disability.

Medication for the treatment of depression

There are no systematic controlled drug trials of treatment of depression in people with ID; therefore, general principles of NICE guidance apply.

The existing literature of case reports and case series suggests that the efficacy and effectiveness of antidepressants in people with ID are very similar to those in the general population:

- The efficacy of selective serotonin reuptake inhibitors (SSRIs) and of tricyclic antidepressants (TCAs) is similar.
- SSRIs are considered to be better tolerated than TCAs. TCAs may have unwanted side effects such as anticholinergic effects, postural hypotension and cardiac conduction disturbances.

Concerns about antidepressants

There are concerns about the widespread prescribing of antidepressants in the ID population. Studies of such prescribing show that the antidepressants are prescribed for a wide range of behaviours and symptoms common in ID rather than for depression. In addition, there are the following problems associated with using antidepressants in people with ID:

- Most antidepressants present a moderate risk of worsening seizures. The risk is lower with SSRIs and monoamine oxidase inhibitors (MAOIs) than with TCAs.
- Hypomania and increased maladaptive behaviours have been shown to emerge in up to a third of patients treated with SSRIs.
- There may be withdrawal problems on discontinuation, particularly with paroxetine.
- Hyponatraemia may be an issue, especially in elderly.

Duration and ending of treatment

It is important to start on a low dose initially and then titrate the dose to the maximum tolerated dose. Monitor for side effects and inform the carers about the potential warning signs about side effects.

The duration of treatment for depression and the strategy for ending treatment should be the same as recommended for the general population:

- For the first episode of depression, maintenance treatment should be given for 6–9 months at the dose of antidepressant used to achieve full recovery.
- For recurrent depression, maintenance treatment should be given for 2–5 years at the dose of antidepressant used to achieve full recovery.
- Antidepressant treatment should be gradually withdrawn over a period of 4–6 weeks using a tapering dose regimen to avoid discontinuation reactions.

Discontinuation reactions

Discontinuation reactions characteristically appear within a few days of stopping treatment and usually resolve within 2–4 weeks. Such reactions may be experienced following cessation of TCAs as well as SSRIs and selective noradrenaline reuptake inhibitors (SNRIs). They are more common following the abrupt cessation of the antidepressant and in particular with paroxetine.

Discontinuation reactions usually consist of influenza-like symptoms (fever, nausea, vomiting, insomnia, headache, sweating) and at times anxiety and agitation. Discontinuation reactions to SSRIs may also include dizziness, vertigo and light-headedness and occasionally sensory symptoms such as paraesthesiae, numbness and the sensation of electric shocks.

Discontinuation reactions can be a key issue following medication withdrawal in people with ID. Changes in behaviour due to discontinuation symptoms should not prompt immediate reinstatement of medication; it is vital to educate carers that resolution will naturally occur between 2 and 4 weeks.

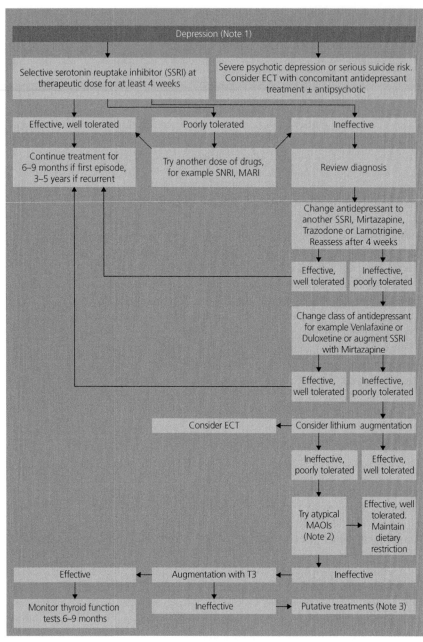

Algorithm 15.1 Treatment of depression in adults with ID.

Treatment of depression in adults with ID

Algorithm 15.1 should be used as a guide only for the treatment of adults with both ID and depression.

Note 1: Drug choice

Drug treatment is indicated for cases with moderate to severe depressive episodes. The choice of drug depends on the presence of any comorbid psychiatric diagnoses (Table 15.1) and whether the person falls into any special group (Table 15.2). The treatment of depression in adults with ID mostly involves using the newer antidepressants because of their reduced incidence of side-effects.

Note 2: Dietary restrictions

There are fewer dietary restrictions with moclobemide than with other MAOls but the restrictions still apply.

Note 3: Putative treatments in resistant depression

The Maudsley Guidelines provides a number of alternatives if first-line treatments remain unsuccessful.

Electroconvulsive therapy

Electroconvulsive therapy (ECT) is recommended only to achieve rapid and short-term improvement of severe symptoms after an adequate trial of other treatment options has proven ineffective and/or when the condition is considered to be potentially life threatening.

A review by Collins et al. (2012) about the use of ECT in people with ID reports that that ECT has been used effectively in this patient population for

Table 15.1 Depression with co-morbid conditions: options for medications.

Co-morbidities	Options for treatment
Depression + symptoms of anxiety	Paroxetine, sertraline, amitriptyline, fluoxetine, trazodone, citalopram, venlafaxine
Depression + psychomotor retardation	Imipramine, fluoxetine, venlafaxine, lofepramine
Depression + obsessive compulsive features	SSRIs, especially paroxetine TCAs, especially clomipramine
Depression + psychotic symptoms	TCAs, probably first drug of choice SSRIs/SNRIs (if TCA poorly tolerated or contraindicated): +/– Small doses of typical or atypical antipsychotics (reasonable evidence for augmentation of an antidepressant with olanzapine or quetiapine) Electroconvulsive therapy if indicated
Depression + deliberate self-harm	SSRIs but avoid citalopram If TCAs are used, then lofepramine is least toxic

Table 15.2 Prescribing in special patient groups.

Special patient groups	Drug choice in depression
Women of childbearing age	SSRIs, especially fluoxetine
Pregnant women	Adequate experience with imipramine and amitriptyline
	And in the SSRIs, especially fluoxetine (risk with fluoxetine is reduced birth weight and preterm birth)
Breastfeeding women	Sertraline, paroxetine, nortriptyline, imipramine
Older persons	SSRIs, especially paroxetine, citalopram, sertraline and venlafaxine
	Avoid TCAs and reboxetine
People with Down syndrome	SSRIs
People with epilepsy	SSRIs
	Consider moclobemide, other MAOIs, reboxetine, tryptophan, agomelatine
	Adjust dose of antiepileptic drug if necessary
	Avoid TCAs
People with cardiovascular problems	SSRIs
	Avoid TCAs, especially dothiepin
People with renal impairment	Avoid lithium
	Sertraline and citalopram
People with hepatic impairment	Imipramine, paroxetine or citalopram

varying psychiatric conditions with few side effects. There are no controlled studies, but of the 72 case reports, almost 58% were for an affective disorder.

There was no reported cognitive decline in any of the case studies.

ECT should be considered when there is a life-threatening depression, a severe depression or a serious suicide risk.

Illustrative case study 15.1

A 40-year-old woman with a moderate degree of intellectual disability was referred to the psychiatric team with a history of irritability, screaming episodes, hitting staff, poor engagement in activities and refusing to visit her parents' home at weekends. Her sleep pattern was disrupted with intermittent waking, and staff also reported recent weight loss.

She is referred by her general practitioner to the local intellectual disability service.

She is reviewed by the psychiatrist in her home along with the community nurse. The staff provide a 4-week history of the above-mentioned symptoms and also report a poor sleep pattern. On further questioning, it becomes apparent that her key worker at day care has been off work unwell for the last month. The psychiatrist also obtained a collateral history from mother regarding premorbid functioning that revealed that she used to be interested in activities and would go to the day centre regularly and also was sociable and interacted well with the other residents. After obtaining history from the staff and the patient and performing a mental state examination of the patient, a diagnosis of a moderate depressive disorder is made. Although the guidelines state that psychological therapies also need to be offered, due to communication difficulties, this was not found to be feasible.

Discussion case study 15.2

Beatrice, a 55-year-old lady with moderate ID and epilepsy, is seen at the day centre facility for a routine 6-month follow-up of her epilepsy by the ID psychiatry team. She takes sodium valproate, and her seizures are well controlled. Her key worker reports that for the last 3 months, Beatrice has been displaying increasing restlessness, irritability and anger at times during her day activities, which is unlike her. She has been staying in a temporary respite facility for the last 6 weeks and has been coming in somewhat unkempt and smelling of body odour for the last 3 weeks. On talking to respite facility staff, it becomes apparent that Beatrice has been unwilling to accept personal care, screaming and appearing agitated when asked to take a shower. The staff have been reluctant to push the issue, as they report that Beatrice's father passed away from a heart attack 4 months ago while taking a bath and was found later by Beatrice and mum.

On questioning, Beatrice is eating and sleeping as normal and continuing to get ready in the mornings to attend her day activities as usual.

Questions
• What is your differential diagnosis?
• What management strategies could be tried if Beatrice has depression?
• What is the potential impact of drug treatment for depression on Beatrice's epilepsy, and how should this be managed?

An SSRI is initiated and community nurses were involved in monitoring mood and side effects, conducting risk assessment and educating staff/mother about depressive disorders and implementing supportive strategies to help the patient.

Key guidance

NICE. (2010) Depression in adults: the NICE guideline on the treatment and management of depression in adults. CG90. http://www.nice.org.uk/guidance/cg90/resources/cg90-depression-in-adults-full-guidance2 (accessed 8 January 2015).

References

Collins J, Halder N, Chaudhry N. (2012) Use of ECT in patients with an intellectual disability: review. *Psychiatric Bulletin* 36:55–60.

Kannabiran M, McCarthy J. (2009) The mental health needs of people with autism spectrum disorders. *Psychiatry* 8:398–401.

Kessing LV. (2007) Epidemiology of subtypes of depression. *Acta Psychiatrica Scandinavica* 115(Suppl. 433):85–89.

Lewinsohn PM, Solomon A, Seeley JR, Zeiss A. (2000) Clinical implications of subthreshold depressive symptoms. *Journal of Abnormal Psychology* 109:345–351.

Turky A, Beavis JM, Thapar AK, Kerr MP. (2008) Psychopathology in children and adolescents with epilepsy: an investigation of predictive variables. *Epilepsy & Behavior* 12:136–144.

Walker JC, Dosen A, Buitelaar JK, Janzing JGE. (2011) Depression in Down syndrome: a review of the literature. *Research in Developmental Disabilities* 32(5):1432–1440.

Further reading

Hurley AD. (2006) Mood disorders in intellectual disability. *Current Opinion in Psychiatry* 19:465–469.

Janowsky DS, Shetty M, Barnhill J, Elamir B, Davis J. (2005) Serotonergic antidepressant effects on aggressive, self-injurious and destructive/disruptive behaviours in intellectually disabled adults: a retrospective, open-label, naturalistic trial. *The International Journal of Neuropsychopharmacology* 8(1):37–48.

Rail PR, Kerr M. (2010) Antidepressant use in adults with intellectual disability. *Psychiatric Bulletin* 34:123–126.

Sohanpal SK, Deb S, Thomas C, Soni R, Lenôtre L, Unwin G. (2007) The effectiveness of anti-depressant medication in the management of behaviour problems in adults with intellectual disabilities: a systematic review. *Journal of Intellectual Disability Research* 51(10):750–765.

Turky A, Felce D, Jones G, Kerr M. (2011) Prospective case control study of psychiatric disorders in adults with epilepsy and intellectual disability. *Epilepsia* 52(7):1223–1230.

Underwood L, McCarthy J, Tsakanikos E. (2010) Mental health of adults with autism spectrum disorders and intellectual disability. *Current Opinion in Psychiatry* 23:421–426.

CHAPTER 16

Bipolar Affective Disorder

Dasari Mohan Michael[1], David Branford[2] & Mary Barrett[3]

[1]*Humber NHS Foundation Trust, East Riding of Yorkshire, UK*
[2]*English Pharmacy Board, Royal Pharmaceutical Society, London, UK*
[3]*Leicestershire Partnership NHS Trust, Leicester, UK*

> Melancholia is the beginning and a part of mania.... The development of a mania is really a worsening of the disease (melancholia) rather than a change into another disease.
> — *Aretaeus of Cappadocia (c. AD 30–90)*

Definition

Bipolar affective disorder is characterised by repeated episodes in which the patient's mood and activity levels are significantly disturbed, with on some occasions an elevation of mood and increased energy and activity (mania or hypomania) and on others a lowering of mood and decreased energy and activity (depression) (SIGN Clinical Guideline 82). The condition is commonly sub-classified as follows:

Bipolar I disorder

One or more manic episodes or mixed episodes.

Individuals often have one or more major depressive episodes.

Bipolar II disorder

One or more major depressive episodes accompanied by at least one hypomanic episode.

Prevalence

The latest evidence suggests that the point prevalence of all affective disorders is 6.6%. Of these, 4.1% were unipolar depressive disorders, 0.5% were bipolar depressive episodes, 0.6% were manic episodes, 1.2% were bipolar disorders, and 0.3% were cyclothymic disorders.

The Frith Prescribing Guidelines for People with Intellectual Disability, Third Edition.
Edited by Sabyasachi Bhaumik, David Branford, Mary Barrett and Satheesh Kumar Gangadharan.
© 2015 John Wiley & Sons, Ltd. Published 2015 by John Wiley & Sons, Ltd.

Clinical presentation

Diagnosis in people with ID can be challenging due to the difficulties arising from communication problems, the influence of poor physical and social circumstances and a general lack of suitable diagnostic criteria. In addition, differences in presenting symptoms such as changes in behaviour, and the need to rely on observable symptoms rather than the person being able to articulate their inner mental state, add to the diagnostic challenge. Thus, the overall prevalence in this population may be underestimated.

Cain et al. (2003) in a retrospective case study stated that bipolar disorder can be readily recognised and distinguished from other behavioural and psychiatric diagnoses in individuals with ID and that DSM-IV criteria can be useful in the diagnosis of bipolar disorder.

Matson et al. (2007) suggested that psychomotor agitation, decreased sleep, changes in mood and aggression were significantly related to the diagnosis of mania. Further, psychomotor agitation and disturbed sleep were significant predictors of a diagnosis of mania. They also suggested that DSM-IV criteria were useful.

Mania and hypomania in ID generally present with an increase in motor activity. Mood is less likely to be euphoric or infectious and more likely to be irritable and accompanied at times by aggression. While pressure of speech may be present, more complex verbal symptoms such as flight of ideas or clang associations are rare. Grandiose ideas and delusions are usually in a simple form; and hallucinations are rare.

Rapid cycling bipolar disorder (four or more episodes of affective illness in 1 year) is associated with severe behaviour problems in individuals with ID, particularly self-injurious behaviour.

Medication for bipolar affective disorder

General recommendations

The patient and carers should be involved as much as possible in decisions about their treatment and care and determine treatment plans in collaboration with the patient and carers, carefully considering the experience and outcome of previous treatment(s) together with patient preference.

Mania/hypomania

If a patient develops acute mania when not taking antimanic medication, treatment options include starting an antipsychotic, valproate or lithium.

When making the choice, prescribers should take into account preferences for future prophylactic use and the side effect profile and consider:

• Prescribing an antipsychotic if there are severe manic symptoms or marked behavioural disturbance as part of the syndrome of mania.

- Prescribing valproate or lithium if symptoms have responded to these medications before and the person has shown good compliance.
- Avoiding valproate in women of childbearing potential.
- Using lithium only if symptoms are not severe because it has a slower onset of action than antipsychotics and valproate.
- Person's likely compliance with drug monitoring (see Table 16.1). Blood testing can prove particularly difficult to achieve in some people with ID.
- In the initial management of acute behavioural disturbance or agitation, the short-term use of a benzodiazepine should be considered in addition to the antimanic agent.

Several antipsychotics have now been licensed for use in the treatment of mania, for example, quetiapine, olanzapine, aripiprazole and risperidone. However, aripiprazole has the additional licence for reoccurrence prevention of mania and quetiapine for prevention of mania in bipolar disorders. If treating acute mania with antipsychotics, the following should be taken into account:

- Individual risk factors for side effects (such as the risk of diabetes).
- The need to initiate treatment at the lower end of the therapeutic dose range recommended in the summary of product characteristics and titrate according to response.
- If an antipsychotic proves ineffective, augmenting it with valproate or lithium should be considered.
- That older people are at greater risk of sudden onset of depressive symptoms after recovery from a manic episode.

Carbamazepine should not be routinely used for treating acute mania, and gabapentin, lamotrigine and topiramate are not recommended.

Medication combinations such as antipsychotics and benzodiazepines are frequently used in clinical practice to control behaviour symptoms associated with mania. Although adjunctive treatment is necessary in many cases, there are risks of misdiagnosing the primary psychiatric disorder and of treatment being used for non-specific behaviour control. The latter may result in excessive use of tranquillising medication, without optimal therapeutic benefit to the patient (Algorithm 16.1).

Algorithm 16.1 should be used as a guide only for the treatment of adults with both ID and first episode of mania or hypomania. This incorporates guidance from NICE on the use of olanzapine and sodium valproate in the treatment of acute mania associated with bipolar disorder.

Note 1: First episode

In the acute treatment of the first episode of mania and hypomania, antipsychotic medication alone or in combination with a benzodiazepine has been found to be effective. Treatment should be given for between six months and a year.

Note 2: Rapid tranquillisation

Rapid tranquilisation may be required during the acute excitement phase. Most mental health trusts have policies for the drug management of acutely

Table 16.1 Suggested list of monitoring requirements in the management of bipolar disorder.

Test or measurement	Monitoring for all patients		Monitoring for specific drugs		
	Initial health check-up	Annual check-up	Antipsychotics	Lithium	Valproate	Carbamazepine
Thyroid function	✓	✓a		At start and every 6 months; more often if evidence of deterioration		
Liver function	✓				At start and at 6 months	At start and at 6 months
Renal function	✓			At start and every 6 months; more often if there is evidence of deterioration or the patient starts taking drugs such as ACE inhibitors, diuretics or NSAIDs		
Full blood count	✓		Only if clinically indicated	At start and once during first 6 months		At start and at 6 months
Blood (plasma glucose)	✓	✓	At start and at 3 months (and at 1 month if taking olanzapine); more often if there is evidence of elevated levels			
Lipid profile	✓	Over 40s only	At start and 3 months; more often if evidence of elevated levels			
Blood pressure	✓	✓				
Prolactin	Children and adolescents only		Risperidone only at start and if symptoms of raised prolactin develop			
ECG	If indicated by history or clinical picture		At start if there are risk factors for or existing cardiovascular disease	At start if there are risk factors for or existing cardiovascular disease		

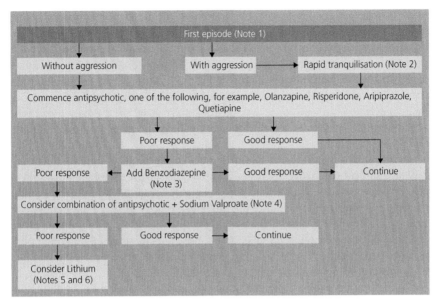

Algorithm 16.1 Treatment of first episode mania and hypomania in adults with ID.

disturbed behaviour (rapid tranquillisation), and local policies should be followed. Rapid tranquillisation usually comprises three stages: firstly, talking therapies, if these are unsuccessful followed secondly by oral drug treatment (usually oral lorazepam, risperidone or olazapine) which, if unsuccessful, is followed thirdly by parenteral (IM) therapies. These parenteral therapies include lorazepam 1–2 mg IM stat either alone or with haloperidol 2–5 mg IM. An alternative is IM olanzapine (alone) 5–10 mg but this must not be given with IM lorazepam. Although rather slow in onset for use in rapid tranquillisation, zuclopenthixol acetate may be a useful adjuvant to consider if the behaviour continues to necessitate a number of IM interventions.

Note 3: Duration of treatment

The use of benzodiazepines should be restricted to 4 weeks to avoid the risk of physical dependency.

Note 4: Combinations of antipsychotic drugs and valproate

Valproate: starting with 200 mg twice a day and gradually increasing the dose according to the response. A wide variety of formulations and brands or sodium valproate and semi-sodium valproate are available.

Note 5: Contraindications to lithium

Lithium is teratogenic and carries a one in 1000 risk of causing Ebstein's anomaly. Whenever possible, it should be avoided during pregnancy, especially in the first trimester. However, the decision to continue to prescribe lithium during pregnancy should be made after weighing the risk of relapse against the risk of causing a foetal abnormality. One option may be to reduce the dose of lithium until the least effective dose is reached. During the later stages of pregnancy, the dose may need to be increased due to the increased maternal renal clearance and fluid volume. Serum lithium levels should be monitored at least once a month throughout pregnancy and more frequently in the third trimester. Adequate water and salt intake must be maintained throughout pregnancy. Thyroid function must be monitored. Patients should be advised to report symptoms of toxicity immediately.

Lithium is contraindicated in Addison's disease and renal or cardiac disease and during lactation.

In people with epilepsy, therapeutic doses of lithium may induce electroencephalogram (EEG) changes. It may also lower the seizure threshold, resulting in generalised tonic–clonic and myoclonic seizures. Co-administration with carbamazepine or phenytoin may predispose to neurotoxicity, which is associated with seizures. It has been found that pre-existing EEG abnormalities, concomitant antipsychotic medication, cerebral pathology and genetic susceptibility predispose to lithium toxicity.

Note 6: Monitoring lithium levels

Serum lithium concentration for prophylaxis is 0.4–0.8 mmol/L, and the dose may be adjusted to achieve this. The optimum dose varies among individuals. During lithium prophylaxis, the serum concentration should be monitored every 2–3 months. Baseline investigations (see following text) should be repeated every 6 months. Lithium prophylaxis should ideally last 3–4 years, but therapy should be continued only if the benefits persist.

Medication treatment of acute mania for people taking antimanic medication

If a patient already taking an antipsychotic experiences a manic episode, the dose should be checked and increased if necessary. If there are no signs of improvement, the addition of lithium or valproate should be considered.

If a patient already taking lithium experiences a manic episode, plasma lithium levels should be checked. If levels are suboptimal (i.e. below 0.8 mmol/L), the dose should normally be increased to a maximum blood level of 1.0 mmol/L. If the response is not adequate, augmenting lithium with an antipsychotic should be considered.

If a patient already taking valproate experiences a manic episode, the dose should be increased until:

• Symptoms start to improve or
• Side effects limit further dose increase

If there are no signs of improvement, the addition of olanzapine, quetiapine, aripiprazole or risperidone should be considered. People with ID on doses higher than 45 mg/kg should be monitored carefully.

For people with ID who present with severe mania when already taking lithium or valproate, adding an antipsychotic should be considered at the same time as gradually increasing the dose of lithium or valproate.

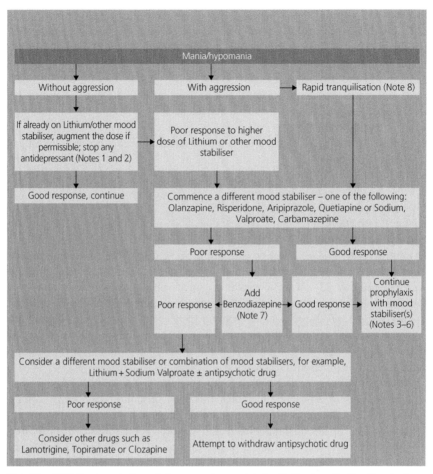

Algorithm 16.2 Treatment of mania/hypomania associated with bipolar affective disorder in adults with ID.

For people with ID who present with mania when already taking carbamazepine, the dose should not routinely be increased. Adding an antipsychotic should be considered, depending on the severity of mania and the current dose of carbamazepine. Interactions with other medication are common with carbamazepine, and doses should be adjusted as necessary.

Algorithm 16.2 should be used as a guide only of the treatment of adults with both ID and suffering from repeated episodes of bipolar affective disorder.

Note 1: Acute treatment

During an acute attack of mania or hypomania, lithium treatment may take 10 days or more to exert its antimanic effect, and therefore, concomitant treatment with a benzodiazepine or antipsychotic drugs is usually required. The dose of antipsychotic drug should be kept low if co-prescribed with lithium because high doses of typical antipsychotics such as haloperidol and fluphenazine or flu-penthixol have been known to cause irreversible toxic encephalopathy when used concomitantly with lithium.

Note 2: Antidepressants

If on an antidepressant, abruptly or gradually reduce and stop depending on the clinical need and risk of withdrawal problems.

Note 3: Prophylaxis

Before beginning treatment with a mood-stabilising drug, baseline investigations should be done:

- Full blood count (FBC)
- Urea and electrolyte (U&E) levels
- Liver function tests (LFTs)
- Thyroid function tests
- Electrocardiogram (ECG)

Lithium treatment should not be started unless serum levels can be monitored. The serum lithium concentration should be measured 1 week after starting treatment and weekly thereafter until the concentration is 0.6–1.0 mmol/L.

Lithium may be started at the same time as an oral antipsychotic, and the antipsychotic stopped at a later date. Alternatively, mood may be initially stabilised using an antipsychotic, and lithium started later, followed by a gradual cessation of the antipsychotic.

Note 4: Monitoring lithium levels

The serum lithium concentration for prophylaxis is 0.4–0.8 mmol/L. The dose of lithium may be adjusted to achieve this. The optimum dose varies among individuals.

During lithium prophylaxis, the serum concentration should be monitored every 2–3 months. The baseline investigations (note 3) should be repeated every 6 months. Lithium prophylaxis should ideally last 3–4 years, but therapy should be continued only if the benefits persist.

Note 5: Other mood-stabilising drugs for prophylaxis

Mood-stabilising drugs used for prophylaxis instead of lithium are:

- Sodium valproate: starting with 200 mg twice a day and gradually increasing the dose according on the response
- Carbamazepine: starting with 100–200 mg/day and gradually increasing the dose according to the response
- Antipsychotic drugs, such as olanzapine, risperidone and quetiapine, for bipolar illness with depressive symptoms as the primary presentation lamotrigine may provide an alternative to antidepressants

Note 6: Contraindications to lithium

Lithium is teratogenic and carries a one in 1000 risk of causing Ebstein's anomaly. Therefore, lithium should whenever possible be avoided during pregnancy, especially in the first trimester. However, the decision to prescribe lithium should be made after weighing the risk of relapse against the risk of causing a foetal abnormality. One option may be to reduce the dose of lithium until the least effective dose is reached. During the later stages of pregnancy, the dose may need to be increased due to the increased maternal renal clearance and fluid volume. Serum lithium levels should be monitored at least once a month throughout pregnancy and more frequently in the third trimester. Adequate water and salt intake must be maintained throughout pregnancy. Thyroid function must be monitored. Patients should be advised to report symptoms of toxicity immediately.

Lithium is contraindicated in Addison's disease, renal or cardiac disease and lactation.

In people with epilepsy, therapeutic doses of lithium may induce EEG changes. It may also lower the seizure threshold, resulting in generalised tonic–clonic and myoclonic seizures. Co-administration with carbamazepine or phenytoin may predispose to neurotoxicity, which is associated with seizures. It has been found that pre-existing EEG abnormalities, concomitant antipsychotic medication, cerebral pathology and genetic susceptibility predispose to lithium toxicity.

Note 7: Duration of treatment

The use of benzodiazepines should be restricted to 4 weeks to avoid the risk of physical dependency.

Note 8: Rapid tranquillisation

Rapid tranquillisation may be required during the acute excitement phase. Most mental health trusts have policies for the drug management of acutely disturbed behaviour (rapid tranquillisation), and local policies should be followed. Rapid tranquillisation usually comprises three stages: firstly, talking therapies, if these are unsuccessful, followed secondly by oral drug treatment (usually oral lorazepam, risperidone or olanzapine), which, if unsuccessful, is followed thirdly by parenteral (IM) therapies. These parenteral therapies include lorazepam 1–2 mg IM stat either alone or with haloperidol 2–5 mg IM. An alternative is IM olanzapine (alone) 5–10 mg, but this must not be given with IM lorazepam. Although rather slow in onset for use in rapid tranquillisation, zuclopenthixol acetate may be a useful adjuvant to consider if the behaviour continues to necessitate a number of IM interventions.

Depression

When treating depressive symptoms in a patient with bipolar disorder in a patient who is not already taking antimanic medication, prescribers should explain the risks of switching to mania and the benefits of taking an adjunctive antimanic agent. Antidepressant treatment should begin at a low dose and be increased gradually if necessary.

If a person has an acute depressive episode when taking antimanic medication, prescribers should first check they are taking the antimanic agent at the appropriate dose and adjust the dose if necessary.

Antidepressants should be avoided for people with ID with depressive symptoms who have:

• Rapid cycling bipolar disorder
• A recent hypomanic episode

Following the remission of depressive symptoms (or symptoms have been significantly less severe for 8 weeks), stopping the antidepressant should be considered to minimise the risks of switching to mania and increased rapid cycling.

Mixed episodes

Mixed episodes of symptoms of mania and depression are not uncommon in people with ID. Prescribers should consider treating people with ID with an acute mixed episode as if they had an acute manic episode, and avoid prescribing an antidepressant and monitor closely.

Illustrative case study 16.1

A 20-year-old man with moderate ID presented to the outpatient clinic with a history of intermittent episodes of challenging behaviour since leaving school at 19 years of age. His parents described that he would periodically present with verbal aggression in the form of shouting and screaming in addition to using abusive language, which was out of character. He would also present at these times as with sexually inappropriate behaviour in the form of touching females and masturbating in public, much to the concern of his parents, which they noted was also out of character. Further history suggested that these symptoms were also associated with disturbances in biological functioning. The apparent trigger was a change in the day-care arrangement.

The psychiatrist completed a full psychiatric assessment including mental state examination, which suggested features of an elated mood, restlessness, pacing, inappropriate touching and apparent lack of inhibitions.

Following the initial assessment, a Psychiatric Assessment Schedule for Adults with Developmental Disability (PAS-ADD) checklist was undertaken by the community nurse, which clearly indicated high scores above the threshold for mania. He was commenced on olanzapine with a working diagnosis of bipolar disorder – current episode mania. Following baseline assessment, he responded initially to olanzapine, but this was not sustained.

A decision was then taken to add a mood stabiliser. Further to baseline investigations, he was commenced on lithium following admission to the inpatient unit since the parents were unable to cope with the aggression at home. A therapeutic level was reached of 0.5 mmol/L at which point he was receiving lithium carbonate 800 mg daily. During the phase of initial titration of lithium, PRN lorazepam was prescribed in order to manage the aggression. By week 4 of the treatment with lithium, his aggression and motor restlessness showed a significant reduction and his biological functions returned to normal. By week 8, he had achieved a premorbid level of functioning and mental state. At subsequent reviews in the outpatient clinic, the dose of olanzapine was gradually reduced and discontinued. He continues to maintain a stable mood and take part in a full programme of activities in the community.

Prophylaxis

Lithium, olanzapine, aripiprazole, quetiapine or valproate should be considered for long-term treatment of bipolar disorder. The choice should depend on:

- Response to previous treatments
- The relative risk, and known precipitants, of manic versus depressive relapse
- Physical risk factors, particularly renal disease, obesity and diabetes
- The patient's preference and history of adherence
- Gender (valproate should not be prescribed for women of childbearing potential)
- A brief assessment of cognitive state (such as the Mini-Mental State Examination) if appropriate, for example, for older people

Lithium has been successfully used in the prophylaxis of bipolar disorder in ID. Lithium is generally well tolerated, although some side effects such as tremors, weight gain and hypothyroidism may be unacceptable. In addition, regular blood monitoring may prove to be difficult in some people with ID due to lack of understanding and co-operation. Other mood-stabilising medications such as carbamazepine and sodium valproate have also been shown to be effective.

If the patient has frequent relapses or symptoms continue to cause functional impairment, switching to an alternative monotherapy or adding a second prophylactic agent (lithium, aripiprazole, quetiapine, olanzapine, valproate) should be considered. Clinical state, side effects and, where relevant, blood levels should be monitored closely. Possible combinations are lithium with valproate, lithium with any of the antipsychotics mentioned above and valproate with any of the antipsychotics mentioned above. The reasons for the choice and the discussion with the patient of the potential benefits and risks should be documented.

If a trial of a combination of prophylactic agents proves ineffective, the following should be considered:

- Carbamazepine: starting with 100–200 mg/day and gradually increasing the dose according to the response
- Consulting with, or referring the patient to, a clinician with expertise in the medication treatment of bipolar disorder
- Prescribing lamotrigine (especially if the patient has bipolar II disorder) or carbamazepine

Long-term medication treatment should normally continue for at least 2 years after an episode of bipolar disorder and up to 5 years if the person has risk factors for relapse, such as a history of frequent relapses or severe psychotic episodes, co-morbid substance misuse, ongoing stressful life events or poor social support.

Rapid cycling

Treatment of rapid cycling bipolar disorder should be as for manic and depressive episodes.

In addition, review the patient's previous treatments for bipolar disorder, and consider a further trial of any that were inadequately delivered or adhered to.

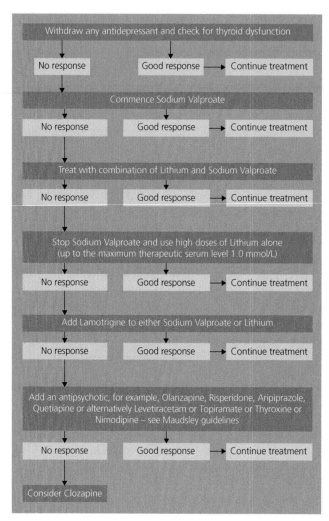

Algorithm 16.3 Treatment of rapid cycling mood disorder in adults with ID.

Focus on long-term treatment, with trials of medication lasting at least 6 months. Algorithm 16.3 illustrates the recommended treatment strategy.

Electroconvulsive therapy

Electroconvulsive therapy (ECT) is recommended only to achieve rapid and short-term improvement of severe symptoms after an adequate trial of other treatment options has proven ineffective and/or when the condition is considered to be potentially life threatening. NICE recommends its usage in individuals with:
- Severe depressive illness (see Chapter 15)
- Catatonia
- A prolonged or severe manic episode

Discussion case study 16.2

Fatima is a 33-year-old lady with a diagnosis of moderate ID and challenging behaviour. Carers report a number of triggers for her behaviour including menstruation, physical ill health (particularly recurrent urine infections) and changes in the family home. She has been treated with risperidone for the past five years with initial benefit; however, her carers now feel this has become ineffective. At your request, carers keep a detailed behaviour record for several months and bring this to the next appointment. The record highlights episodes of agitation, restlessness, irritability, reduced sleep and appetite, associated with self-injury and aggression. The record highlights some relationship with the reported triggers; however, other episodes have no clear trigger.
- What are the diagnostic possibilities?
- What are the treatment options?
- What factors might influence the choice of mood stabiliser in this lady?

Practitioners must be aware of the risk of manic switch if used for a depressive episode.

Monitoring requirements

Table 16.1 summarises the monitoring requirements for the different drug choices discussed. Compliance with testing needs to be considered when choosing between different treatment options.

Key resources

National Institute for Health and Care Excellence (NICE). (2006) Bipolar disorder: the management of bipolar disorder in adults, children and adolescents, in primary and secondary care (CG38). London: NICE.

References

Cain NN, Davidson PW, Burhan AM, et al. (2003) Identifying bipolar disorders in individuals with intellectual disability. *Journal of Intellectual Disability Research* 47(1):31–38.

Cooper S, Smiley E, Morrison J, Williamson A, Allan L. (2007) Mental ill-health in adults with intellectual disabilities: prevalence and associated factors. *The British Journal of Psychiatry* 190:27–35.

Craft M, Ismail IA, Krishnamurti D, et al. (1987) Lithium in the treatment of aggression in mentally handicapped patients: a double-blind trial. *British Journal of Psychiatry* 150:685–689.

Matson JL, González ML, Terlonge C, Thorson RT, Laud RB. (2007) What symptoms predict the diagnosis of mania in persons with severe/profound intellectual disability in clinical practice? *Journal of Intellectual Disability Research* 51(Pt 1):25–31.

CHAPTER 17

Schizophrenia

Avinash Hiremath[1], Amala Jovia Maria Jesu[1], Rohit Gumber[1] & Saduf Riaz[2]

[1]*Leicestershire Partnership NHS Trust, Leicester, UK*
[2]*NHS Greater Glasgow and Clyde, Glasgow, UK*

> Please hear this: There are not 'schizophrenics.'
> There are people with schizophrenia.
>
> *Elyn Saks*

Definition

Schizophrenia is characterised by distortions of thinking and perception together with a blunted or inappropriate affect. Diagnosis requires symptoms to be present for at least a month. Diagnosis is excluded in the presence of organic brain disorder or drug intoxication/withdrawal.

Prevalence

The prevalence of schizophrenia in the general population is between 2.5 and 5.3 per 1000. In the intellectual disability (ID) population, the prevalence of schizophrenia depends on the nature of the study sample and has commonly been quoted at around 3%. Cooper et al. (2007) reported a point prevalence of 4.4% for psychotic disorder, and Morgan et al. (2008) reported the prevalence of schizophrenia among individuals with an ID was at least three times higher than population lifetime estimates and it was also higher than the commonly quoted estimate of 3% for schizophrenia.

Cognitive deficit involving several domains (verbal memory and learning, spatial working memory, attention, speed of information processing, performance IQ and motor skills) has been identified as a widely shared characteristic of schizophrenia in a comprehensive quantitative review. In the absence of overt

The Frith Prescribing Guidelines for People with Intellectual Disability, Third Edition.
Edited by Sabyasachi Bhaumik, David Branford, Mary Barrett and Satheesh Kumar Gangadharan.
© 2015 John Wiley & Sons, Ltd. Published 2015 by John Wiley & Sons, Ltd.

psychotic symptomatology, it can be difficult to tease out what is ID and what is psychosis, and clinicians need to be mindful of the potential for diagnostic overshadowing.

Evidence suggests a potential common aetiology for ID and schizophrenia in a significant proportion of cases. It has also been suggested that people with a dual diagnosis of schizophrenia and ID suffer a greater severity of illness manifestation.

The prevalence of schizophrenia is reported to be highest in those with a mild degree of ID.

The reason for this remains unclear at this stage but may be contributed to by several factors, including the nature of brain damage and diagnostic challenges clinicians face in people with severe to profound ID.

Key points specific to ID

	Key points specific to ID
Atypical presentations	Schizophrenia may manifest atypically in people with ID. Meta-analysis indicates that people with ID experience more negative symptoms than the general population. Those with predominantly negative symptoms may present with a regression of their skills and symptoms such as lack of motivation. These features may be difficult to identify, particularly in those who are recipients of passive care. If positive symptoms predominate, the individual is likely to suffer from simple hallucinations, for example, in the form of noises. Similarly, delusional beliefs tend to have simple themes that are somewhat fantastic. Individuals with a limited ability to communicate may present with hallucinatory behaviour or with extremely disturbed behaviour that is out of character for them
Limited language skills	It is difficult to diagnose schizophrenia reliably in people with limited language skills although diagnosis may be easier in those with a mild degree of ID if sufficient allowance is made for their reduced vocabulary. As the ICD-10, DSM-V and DC-LD systems are all based on language, a diagnosis of schizophrenia is unlikely to be made with confidence in individuals with an IQ of less than 50
Challenging behaviour	Many individuals with ID may have a concomitant behaviour disorder, which may confound a diagnosis of schizophrenia, and this is particularly the case when major impairment of social interaction is a valid criterion
Affective disorders and negative symptoms	Affective disorders are not uncommon in people with ID and schizophrenia. Depression, side effects of antipsychotic drugs and the primary cause of ID itself may prevent a confident diagnosis of negative symptoms
Schizophrenia and autism	Several symptoms of autism overlap with the negative symptoms of schizophrenia, and failure to consider this may lead to inappropriate assignment of diagnoses. Similarities have been explored and include overlap in symptoms of social dysfunction, social interaction and communication, as well as repetitive stereotyped behaviours

	Key points specific to ID
Schizophrenia and epilepsy	About 20–30% of individuals with ID and schizophrenia also have concomitant epilepsy. It may be difficult to make a clinical diagnosis of schizophrenia confidently, especially in the presence of post-ictal symptoms. Similarly, there is considerable overlap between affective and the negative symptoms of schizophrenia and issues related to side effects of anticonvulsant drugs and by the primary cause of the ID. Symptoms of schizophrenia seen peri-ictally and post-ictally, especially those in temporal lobe epilepsy, need to be differentiated from those associated with inter-ictal schizophrenia. Phenomena such as kindling, forced normalisation and lowering of seizure threshold may all be observed
Monitoring progress and response to treatment	Rating scales such as the Clinical Interview Schedule, Psychopathology Inventory for Mentally Retarded Adults (PIMRA) and Diagnostic Assessment for the Severely Handicapped (DASH) can be used; however, these rely on carer information that may not be robust when following up response to treatment in those with ID. In addition, difficulties in monitoring illness progression may be complicated by clinician bias and unreliable assessments of the dose and duration of medication. The PAS-ADD is a more robust tool to inform clinical judgement, for assessment purposes, and can be repeated to assist in monitoring progress

Management

The National Institute for Clinical Excellence has produced guidelines for the core interventions in the treatment of schizophrenia in the general population. The following guidance is based on these recommendations with adaptations for use in the ID population. Clinicians should evaluate the tolerance and efficacy of current treatments against new antipsychotics as they become available.

Side effects

People with ID are more likely to develop side effects with antipsychotics than the general adult population due to their underlying brain damage. Neurological side effects are most common, particularly extrapyramidal effects such as Parkinsonism, dystonia, akathisia (restlessness), tardive dyskinesia and rarely neuroleptic malignant syndrome. However, some abnormal neurological movements may present premorbidly in some individuals due to their underlying brain damage. Therefore, it is important to assess for neurological side effects prior to commencing/changing antipsychotic treatment and to routinely monitor for neurological side effects on a regular basis using scales such as the Abnormal Involuntary Movement Scale (AIMS). People with ID are also likely to experience other side effects such as QTc prolongation, hepatic impairment and blood dyscrasias due to their multi-system impairment, and clinicians need to be aware of such problems and monitor for them on a routine basis. Monitoring for side effects relies on carer involvement, both in education to increase awareness of side effects and to provide support for the individual in undertaking any necessary monitoring investigations. Monitoring by periodic investigations may prove difficult in some individuals due to their lack of understanding and co-operation. Support from the community team to work with the individual and their carer around access issues and the use of strategies such as desensitisation can be helpful in these situations.

It is recommended that an ECG is carried out prior to commencing antipsychotic medication if a specific cardiovascular risk has been identified or they are being admitted as an inpatient. Baseline monitoring of diabetes, lipid profile, blood pressure and weight is recommended (see Chapter 3 for further guidance on physical monitoring). This should be followed by repeat monitoring at 3 months and then annually (more frequently if olanzapine or clozapine; see Taylor et al., 2012).

Cognition

There is good evidence in adults with normal intelligence that antipsychotics may cause sedation, psychomotor impairment and a decreased ability to concentrate. These effects may be compounded in adults with ID because of their underlying organic condition.

Illustrative case study 17.1

Joshua is a 30-year-old man with mild ID. He lives with his mother but can take care of his basic needs and go out on his own. His speech is good but he has hearing impairment and wears hearing aids. He has been on medication for a long time for a diagnosis of psychotic illness made at the age of 21. At times, he refuses to take his medication and becomes irritable and isolates himself. He has recently become erratic at taking his medication again and was found to be carrying a knife. When asked, Joshua stated that there are people following him and he is carrying the knife to protect himself. Further exploration of symptoms revealed that he was also hearing voices of people telling him that they are going to harm him. It also emerged that he was non-compliant with prescribed antipsychotic medication due to difficulties remembering to take his tablets and side effects in the form of tremors and dyskinetic movements. Following a review, his antipsychotic medication was changed to a second-generation drug, and there was also a discussion around the use of depot medication. The community nurse worked closely to improve compliance and educate Joshua on the consequences of non-compliance. With adequate information sharing, using accessible leaflets on medication, Joshua agreed to switch to depot medication so he does not have to remember to take his tablets.

Drug interactions

Co-morbidity such as a physical illness or epilepsy often results in multiple drug regimens for the majority of people with ID. This increases their risk of drug interactions. Some of the important drug interactions are given in Table 17.1. The British National Formulary (BNF) should be consulted for more detailed information.

Table 17.1 Common drug interactions in people with ID being treated for schizophrenia.

Drug combination	Common interactions
Antipsychotics + lithium	Increased risk of EPSEs and possible neurotoxicity when clozapine, flupenthixol, haloperidol, phenothiazines or zuclopenthixol is given with lithium
Antipsychotics + antiepileptics	The threshold for convulsions may be lowered, due to the influence of the antipsychotic drug
	Carbamazepine accelerates the metabolism (i.e. reduces the plasma concentration) of aripiprazole, haloperidol, chlorpromazine, olanzapine, quetiapine, risperidone and paliperidone
	Phenytoin and phenobarbital accelerate the metabolism (i.e. reduces the plasma concentration) of haloperidol, clozapine and aripiprazole
	Lamotrigine reduces the plasma concentration of aripiprazole and quetiapine and increases plasma concentration of olanzapine
	The risk of neutropenia is increased if olanzapine is given with sodium valproate
	The risk of haematological side effects is increased if clozapine is given with carbamazepine
Antipsychotics + antidepressants	Increased risk of arrhythmias with tricyclic antidepressants
	Selective serotonin reuptake inhibitors and venlafaxine increase the plasma concentration of clozapine and haloperidol
	Fluoxetine increases the plasma concentration of clozapine, haloperidol, risperidone and zuclopenthixol
	Increased risk of anti-muscarinic side effects when phenothiazines and clozapine given with tricyclics

Cautionary note

Ideally, only one antipsychotic should be prescribed at any given time, and it is generally unacceptable for more than two antipsychotics to be prescribed concurrently. However, if two antipsychotics are required, the rationale for such a prescription should be clearly documented in the patient's notes. The patient should be monitored regularly for side effects and for the effects of drug interactions. If the prescription of more than two classes of psychotropic medication is considered necessary, a second opinion is advisable.

Drug treatment of schizophrenia and other psychotic disorders in adults with ID (Algorithm 17.1)

Note 1: High-dose antipsychotic use

The Royal College of Psychiatrists produced a consensus statement in 2006 on the use of high-dose antipsychotic medication. Advice about using antipsychotics above the doses in the BNF has been provided by the Royal College of Psychiatrists.

Note 2: Anticholinergics

Anticholinergic drugs should not be prescribed for more than 4 weeks. If the patient requires anticholinergics on a regular basis or for longer than 4 weeks, it

Summary of key recommendations

- High doses of antipsychotic drugs should only be considered after evidence-based strategies have failed and as a carefully monitored therapeutic trial.
- The decision to prescribe high dose (of either an individual agent or through combination) should be taken explicitly and should involve an individual risk–benefit assessment by a fully trained psychiatrist. This should be undertaken in consultation with the wider clinical team and the patient and a patient advocate, if available, and if the patient wishes their presence.
- The decision to prescribe high dose should be documented in the case notes, including the risks and benefits of the strategy, the aims and when and how the outcome will be assessed.
- Dose escalation should be in relatively small increments and allow adequate time for response, and this includes prescribing once the high-dose threshold has been passed. The maximum tolerated dose may be given for at least 3 to 4 weeks before changing the drug.
- The use of PRN medication should be kept under regular review.
- The possible contraindications to high dose for the drug(s) in the patient concerned should be considered before prescribing a high dose.
- Consider possible drug interactions when prescribing high-dose antipsychotic medication.
- Before prescribing high-dose antipsychotics, carry out an ECG to establish a baseline and exclude cardiac contraindications, including long QT syndromes. An ECG should be repeated after a few days and then every 1–3 months in the early stages of high-dose treatment. The ECG should be repeated as clinically indicated. If an ECG cannot be carried out due to lack of patient co-operation, this should be documented in the patient's notes.
- In treatment-resistant psychosis, evidence-based strategies for treatment resistance should be exhausted, including use of clozapine, before resorting to a high dose of antipsychotic medication.

The use of high dose should be treated as a limited therapeutic trial in treatment-resistant schizophrenia, and the dose reduced back to conventional levels after a 3-month period unless the clinical benefits outweigh the risks.

may indicate persistent drug side effects and warrant either a change in dose or choice of drug. In principle, it is not clinically acceptable if a patient being treated with an atypical antipsychotic still needs anticholinergics and the clinician should consider switching to an alternative atypical drug.

If extrapyramidal side effects (EPSEs) of an antipsychotic are severe, it is preferable to change the medication to one better tolerated than to treat with anticholinergics. Anticholinergics should be withdrawn gradually.

Note 3: Efficacy of antipsychotics

Atypical antipsychotics are considered to be as effective as typical antipsychotics in the treatment of positive symptoms. Clozapine has been found to be effective in the treatment of refractory psychosis and negative symptoms. Risperidone, quetiapine, amisulpride and olanzapine have also been found to be useful in the treatment of negative symptoms. The choice of drug should be made after considering side effects including EPSEs, metabolic side effects and other side effects.

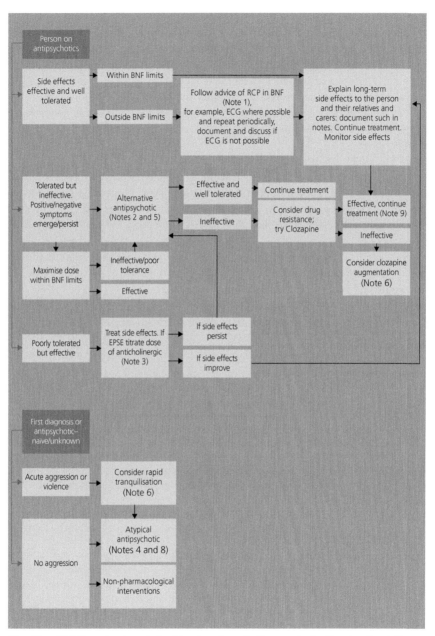

Algorithm 17.1 Drug treatment of schizophrenia and other psychotic disorders in adults with ID.

Note 4: Switching antipsychotics

There is no consensus on how to switch antipsychotics. It should be noted that antipsychotics may produce gastric side effects, particularly those with inherent muscarinic activity. Many antipsychotics have long elimination half-lives, particularly in depot formulation; and switches may take many weeks or months. The BNF provides guidance of equivalent doses when making a switch. Knowledge of the side effect profiles of various antipsychotics should enable effective switching if drugs are not tolerated. Consider depot antipsychotic medication if non-adherence is an issue.

Note 5: Augmentation strategies

Augmentation strategies include lithium for schizo-affective symptoms, carbamazepine for aggression and sodium valproate for mood disturbance. Consider clozapine if no response to two different antipsychotics. Clozapine should not be used concurrently with carbamazepine due to haematological side effects and drug interactions.

If augmentation strategies fail, consider unproven therapies (poor evidence based and increased side effects) such as the following:
Clozapine and sulpiride

Table 17.2 Drug treatment of schizophrenia in special patient groups.

Special patient groups	Drug choice in schizophrenia
Pregnant women	• *Avoid* all antipsychotics in the first trimester if possible • Most experience is with chlorpromazine, haloperidol and trifluoperazine • Olanzapine is widely used by perinatal services in the UK • *Avoid* risperidone and amisulpride if hyperprolactinaemia is symptomatic
Lactating women	• *Avoid* all antipsychotics unless absolutely necessary • Chlorpromazine appears to be safest but causes drowsiness in the infant • Sulpiride and olanzapine considered best choices if medication necessary
Young and middle-aged men and women	• Olanzapine, risperidone, quetiapine or amisulpride • Monitor weight gain and hyperprolactinaemia, particularly with risperidone and amisulpride • *Avoid* risperidone and amisulpride if hyperprolactinaemia is symptomatic • Use quetiapine for those who have acute dystonia or other EPSEs with other antipsychotics
Older men and women	• Olanzapine, risperidone or amisulpride in low doses • Begin slowly and increase slowly while monitoring side effects frequently NB: Committee on Safety of Medicines warning – there is an increased risk of cerebrovascular adverse events in older patients with schizophrenia when treated with olanzapine, or risperidone, quetiapine and aripiprazole
Obese men and women	• *Avoid* olanzapine, clozapine and chlorpromazine • Prefer the use of aripiprazole or amisulpride
People with epilepsy	• Amisulpride, aripiprazole, haloperidol, trifluoperazine and risperidone are preferred choices • Olanzapine, quetiapine and sulpiride probably safe • Avoid chlorpromazine and clozapine if possible • Depot preparations to be used with extreme care

Clozapine and aripiprazole
Clozapine and small doses of risperidone or amisulpride or haloperidol
A course of electroconvulsive therapy

The patient's consent should be gained wherever possible. Therapy should be documented in the patient's notes and continued for a fixed period of 3–4 weeks with frequent evaluation.

Note 6: Special patient groups

Compared with typical antipsychotics, patients on atypical antipsychotics are at a lower risk of short-term side effects in the form of acute EPSEs, although some atypical drugs have a cleaner profile in this regard than others. Even at low doses of antipsychotics, older people are more likely to develop extrapyramidal symptoms, particularly with typical antipsychotics. Long-term use of atypical antipsychotics can have metabolic side effects. These characteristics should be taken into consideration when prescribing to particular patient groups (Table 17.2).

Note 7: Duration of treatment

The duration of treatment depends on patient response. Following the first episode, treatment should be for at least a 2-year symptom-free period ideally with one antipsychotic medication.

Illustrative case study 17.2

Ayesha is 23 years old and has lived in a residential home for the last 5 years. She has moderate ID and epilepsy. She can use words and some short sentences. She can indicate her needs but requires assistance with personal care. Carers have to speak slowly and repeat words to communicate with her. She was referred to the local ID psychiatrist following episodes of disturbed behaviour over the past few weeks. She presents with periods of getting agitated and irritable with poor sleep and appetite. On occasions, she also ran out of her bedroom saying that there is a 'cat', and she can be extremely frightened in these situations.

The psychiatrist completed a full psychiatric assessment, with involvement and support from the community nursing team. Collateral information was obtained from carers and family members who indicated that this behaviour is out of character for her and not typical of/occurring with her seizures. There is a family history of schizophrenia in her maternal aunt. The nurse carried out a series of behavioural observations in the residential home and the day centre to identify specific antecedents, but no particular trigger was present. Physical examination was normal and baseline bloods and ECG were in the normal range. A diagnosis of first episode psychosis was made, and an intervention package designed, with input from various members of the MDT.

Ayesha responded well to cautious introduction of amisulpride (see Table 17.1), which was prescribed at a low dose and gradually titrated with close monitoring for side effects and impact on seizure control. The carers were provided information on expected benefits and possible side effects, and the community nurse visited regularly during the initial stages of treatment. Ayesha quickly showed a reduction in agitation, associated with improved sleep and better engagement at day centre. Within a month, she had stopped reporting seeing the cat, and after a few months on treatment, her behaviour settled completely.

Discussion case study 17.3

> Charles is a 25-year-old man with mild ID. He has lived in a residential home for the past 7 years. Normally, he is a pleasant person who can travel independently. He has a stammer but can otherwise communicate reasonably.
>
> Recently, he started to be irritable with staff and withdrawn and his smoking considerably increased. A few days later, he started sitting in the lounge through the night, watching movies and turning up the volume. He subsequently became physically aggressive and appeared to be talking to an unseen stimulus, when observed by staff. There is a history of some 'mental health problems' in his mother. In the past, Charles has 'got in with the wrong crowd' and used cannabis but denies current use. He is referred by the GP to ID psychiatry services for further assessment.
>
> Questions
> - What are the diagnostic possibilities?
> - What would be treatment options in terms of medication?
> - What other management strategies could be used?

References

Cooper SA, Smiley E, Morrison J, Williamson A, Allan L. (2007) Mental ill-health in adults with intellectual disabilities: prevalence and associated factors. *The British Journal of Psychiatry* 190:27–35.

Morgan VA, Leonard H, Bourke J, Jablensky A. (2008) Intellectual disability co-occurring with schizophrenia and other psychiatric illness: population-based study. *The British Journal of Psychiatry* 193:364–372.

Taylor D, Paton C, Kapur S. (2012) *The Maudsley prescribing guidelines in psychiatry.* 11th edition. London: Wiley-Blackwell.

Further reading

Duggan L, Brylewski J. (1998) Antipsychotic medication for those with both schizophrenia and learning disability (Cochrane review). In: *Cochrane library, Issue 3,* Oxford: Update Software.

Duggan L, Brylewski J. (1999) Effectiveness of antipsychotic medication in people with intellectual disability and schizophrenia: a systematic review. *Journal of Intellectual Disability Research* 43:94–104.

Michael J. (2012) Owen intellectual disability and major psychiatric disorders: a continuum of neurodevelopmental causality. *The British Journal of Psychiatry* 200:268–269.

National Institute for Health and Care Excellence. (2009) Schizophrenia: core interventions in the treatment and management of schizophrenia in adults in primary and secondary. NICE guidance CG 82. www.nice.org.uk/cg82 (accessed 8 January 2015).

Palucka AM, Bradley E, Lunsky Y. (2008, April) A case of unrecognized intellectual disability and autism misdiagnosed as schizophrenia: are there lessons to be learned? *Mental Health Aspects of Developmental Disabilities.*

Welch KA, Lawrie SM, Muir W, Johnstone EC. (2011) Systematic review of the clinical presentation of schizophrenia in intellectual disability. *Journal of Psychopathology and Behavioral Assessment* 33(2):246–253.

CHAPTER 18

Alcohol Use Disorders

Helen Miller

National Deaf Service, South West London and St Georges Mental Health NHS Trust, Springfield University Hospital, London, UK

The growth of 'substance misuse' in both the general and psychiatric populations appears to be mirrored in a growing trend for people with intellectual disabilities who also hazardously use alcohol and drugs.

Taggart et al. (2006)

Definition

Alcohol consumption occurs along a continuum with no clear demarcation between 'social' and 'problem' drinking. As the average amount of drinking and of intoxication increases, so do associated medical and psychosocial problems. Alcohol use disorders are defined in ICD-10 (WHO) as 'acute intoxication', 'harmful use' and 'dependence syndrome'. 'Harmful use' is a pattern of drinking that has already caused damage to health, either physical or psychiatric, but does not meet the criteria for dependence.

DIAGNOSIS OF DEPENDENCE

At least three criteria are present during the past 12 months out of:
- A compulsion to drink
- Withdrawal
- Tolerance
- Impaired control of drinking
- Neglect of alternative interests
- Continued use despite harmful consequences to health

The Frith Prescribing Guidelines for People with Intellectual Disability, Third Edition.
Edited by Sabyasachi Bhaumik, David Branford, Mary Barrett and Satheesh Kumar Gangadharan.

Clinical presentation

Table 18.1 lists the common clinical presentations of alcohol use disorders in people with ID.

Adults with ID who are male and young, who have mild to borderline IQs and mental health problems (including ADHD) and who live alone are particularly vulnerable to developing alcohol use disorders. People with ID are also vulnerable to a number of factors, which have been shown to be risk factors for developing alcohol use disorders in the general population. Table 18.2 lists these.

Illustrative case study 18.1

> Tom has mild ID and a mood disorder and is on prescribed medication, which is administered by staff in his group home. He binge drinks, and when binge drinking, he neglects his self-care, experiences erratic mood swings and has thoughts of self-harm. During alcohol binges, he has damaged his bedroom, been aggressive and oppositional to staff, self-harmed and taken overdoses of painkillers and has had to attend A&E while intoxicated. On one occasion, he refused to go to hospital after taking an overdose of painkillers and was aggressive and threatening to the paramedics who attended him at home.
>
> Ruth has moderate ID and lives at home with her family but after the death of a beloved niece started to drink increasing amounts of alcohol. She now refuses to attend the day centre and spends all day in the local park drinking with her new group of 'friends'. Her community ID team are concerned her new 'friends' are transient alcohol and drug misusers who are exploiting her financially. Her family report rows at home and that she stays out through the night.
>
> Paul has mild ID and paranoid schizophrenia. He experienced a deprived and abusive childhood. He lives alone and is very socially isolated. He goes out to buy alcohol and then stays in drinking while watching TV. He does not wash and often does not answer the door to members of the community team. He has run out in the street shouting and waving a knife when intoxicated and is a victim of bullying from local children.

Prevalence

Table 18.3 lists the prevalence of alcohol use disorders at different levels of ability (from Cooper et al., 2007).

Assessment

The management of alcohol use disorders begins with accurate recognition and diagnosis. Simply asking people if they drink and how much is not enough to determine whether they are drinking in harmful quantities. The Single Alcohol Screening Questionnaire (SASQ) involves asking, 'When was the last time you had 6/8 units (6 for women and 8 for men) of alcohol on any one occasion?' An answer of 'Sometime within the last 3 months' indicates a positive score, and the person and carer should receive brief information and advice.

Table 18.1 Common clinical presentations of alcohol use disorders in ID.

Presentation	Key associations
Aggression	• Verbal aggression more common than physical aggression • Physical aggression to carers, other service users or public • Violent behaviours • Links with conduct disorder and ADHD, especially if co-occurring • Destruction of property
Mental health problems	• Suicidal ideation when drinking • Erratic mood changes • More likely to have co-morbid mental health problem especially psychosis or mood disorder
Risk behaviours	• Suicide attempts • Self-injury • Accidents and injuries, especially road traffic accidents • Fighting • Sexually risky behaviours
Exploitation	• Sexual, physical, financial and psychological • Females particularly vulnerable • Females may make claims of sexual harassment against unknown males while intoxicated
Difficulty maintaining relationships	• Rows with carers and family members • Problems maintaining positive relationships • Poor social judgement • May cut off from carers and family members critical of their drinking and prefer to socialise with others who have alcohol use disorders • Friendships may be unequal with person with ID being exploited financially or sexually
Loss of daily routine	• Poor attendance at activities such as day centre, college or supported employment • Loss of motivation and co-operation • May become socially isolated • May neglect self-care and care of accommodation
Use of other substances	• Smoking most common • Smoking in adolescents who have ADHD, especially if co-morbid conduct disorder, is a red flag for development of alcohol use disorder • Combining alcohol use with combinations of illicit medication use and prescribed medications
Physical health problems	• Attendance at emergency department under influence of alcohol • Increased epileptic activity • Increased rates of sensory disability compared to general ID population • Sexually acquired diseases and HIV • Cardiovascular, respiratory and gastrointestinal and neurological problems • Self-neglect and poor diet • Hard to engage in health education and promotion activities • Poor dentition and oral hygiene
Contact with police/law	• Link with offending behaviours • Link with admission to special hospitals • Antisocial behaviours and shoplifting common offences • Males more than females

Table 18.2 Risk factors for developing alcohol use disorders.

Risk factor	Description
Psychiatric illness	• There is a higher prevalence of alcohol use disorders in people with psychiatric illnesses than the general population (between 8 and 15% in community and in up to 49% of inpatients) • People with ID have a higher prevalence of psychiatric illness than the general population • When alcohol use disorders occur in adults with mental illness, there is a more rapid transition from use to abuse and to dependence • Adults with ID who misuse alcohol have been found to have high rates of mental health problems (39% in one community sample) • Either the alcohol use disorder or the psychiatric illness may be primary, resulting in subsequent development of the other, or they may occur as dual primary diagnoses
Experiences of sexual abuse	• People with ID are vulnerable to sexual abuse • In the general population, adults with histories of sexual abuse have an increased rate of alcohol use disorders • When compared to subjects with alcohol use disorders who have not been abused, subjects with histories of sexual abuse tend to be younger, start drinking younger and have family histories of alcohol misuse and to have more alcohol-related problems
Poverty and social exclusion	• These are risk factors for alcohol use, and people with ID are vulnerable to both
ADHD	• This is a major risk factor for development of alcohol use disorders especially if there is co-morbid conduct disorder • ADHD predicts an earlier age of alcohol use disorder onset, more rapid transition from use to abuse and dependence and longer duration of alcohol use disorder

When asking people with ID about units, it is a good idea to ask them what they drink. Ask them to show you the drink they are referring to, for example, ask them to keep empty bottles or cans to show you. Then ask how much of this drink do they drink at any one time; the number of units can then be calculated. Adults with ID find the concept of units difficult, and pictorial representations can be

ASSESSMENT OF ALCOHOL USE SHOULD COVER THE FOLLOWING AREAS:

Alcohol use including:
  Consumption (historical and recent patterns of drinking,
    use a drinking diary, collateral information)
  Dependence
  Alcohol-related problems
Other medication uses
Physical health
Psychological and social problems
Cognitive function (any evidence of change)
Understanding of alcohol and its effects and readiness to change

Table 18.3 Prevalence of alcohol use disorders in ID.

IQ level	Prevalence (%)		
	Men	**Women**	**Total**
Mild	2.5	1.0	1.8
Moderate to profound	0.8	0.0	0.5
All levels of IQ	1.4	0.4	1.0

Illustrative case study 18.2

Ben has mild ID and lives in temporary accommodation. He started to drink heavily after the death of his more able partner. He was unable to cope and was evicted by his landlord after falling behind in his rent and allowing homeless people he met on the street and regarded as friends to stay in his flat resulting in significant damage to the property. He came to the attention of ID services after he tried to jump off a bridge.

The ID team liaised with the local alcohol team, and after a 4-week inpatient detoxification programme at the alcohol service, he is discharged on an SSRI and is followed up by a counsellor from the community alcohol team and the ID team. The ID team help him find permanent accommodation and outreach support, which works with him to support him with activities of daily living and to rebuild his social network and to move away from the friends he met on the street who tend to borrow money from him and encourage him to drink. After a year, he starts to talk about the emotional impact of the loss of his partner and begins bereavement counselling.

helpful. Collateral histories from family and professional carers are invaluable when obtaining an alcohol history.

Management

Treatment goals vary with the severity of alcohol use disorder (Table 18.4). For harmful drinking and mild dependence without significant co-morbidity and if there is good social support, return to a safe level of drinking may be acceptable. For people with severe alcohol dependence or those who misuse alcohol and have significant psychological or physical co-morbidity, abstinence is the ideal, but if they are unwilling to consider abstinence, consider harm reduction while working with them to encourage them to consider abstinence.

Active involvement of family and carers in the management plan and treatment strategies is important in all cases.

Role of medication

Medication is used to alleviate withdrawal symptoms and to stop them from progressing to more serious symptoms, for example, delirium tremens. Benzodiazepines and antiepileptics are the most commonly used medications.

Table 18.4 Management of alcohol use disorders in adults with ID.

Action	Description
1. Identification	• Ask all users and carers about alcohol use • Be aware of high-risk groups • Look out for alcohol-associated behavioural or physical problems • Use questionnaires (e.g. SASQ) together with pictures to illustrate units of alcohol
2. Brief intervention	• Give simple advice on what is safe to drink, for example, no more than three drinks a day and have three abstinence days a week • Support verbal advice with appropriate literature
3. Joint working with community alcohol teams	• Community alcohol teams assess the person and their addiction and devise a programme and allocate a key worker. They have good links with local voluntary organisations • Community alcohol teams may assume too high a pre-existing knowledge about alcohol in adults with ID, and their programmes and group work may start at too difficult a level, and written materials may be inaccessible for adults with ID • ID teams can support the community alcohol team on issues relevant to ID
4. Managing withdrawal	• The objectives are relief of discomfort, prevention or treatment of complications and preparation for rehabilitation • Diagnose and treat coexisting medical problems (full physical examination and check liver function and full blood count) • Check urea and electrolytes and be aware fluid and electrolyte repletion may be needed • Thiamine (50–100 mg/day oral or IM) and multivitamins prevent the development of alcohol-related neurological disturbance
5. Mild or moderate withdrawal	• May not need medication treatment • Treat with reassurance and attention, monitoring vital signs, reality orientation and nursing care
6. More serious withdrawal reactions	• Inpatient detoxification and medication treatment are needed in people who: – Have serious medical or surgical illnesses – Have past history of adverse withdrawal reactions – Have current evidence of more serious withdrawal reactions – Drink over 30 units of alcohol a day or between 15 and 20 units and have significant psychiatric or physical co-morbidities and/or a learning disability
7. Consider the person with ID's ability and support when planning care	• Do they live by themselves? • Do they have additional health problems or mobility problems? • How confident are you in the accuracy of their history? • How competent are they in seeking help especially in an emergency? • Would they be able to differentiate normal mild withdrawal from more serious problems they should seek help for?
8. Antiepileptics	• Check medication blood levels
9. Alcohol dependence	• Consider medications to reduce craving
10. Motivational interviewing	• A powerful cognitive behavioural technique to deal with ambivalence in people with alcohol use disorders • It uses a cyclical model to describe phases of motivation • The person draws up a balance sheet of the pros and cons of receiving treatment and recognises and tackles ambivalence and anticipating relapse • Has been successfully adapted for adults with ID in forensic settings resulting in increases in motivation, self-efficacy and determination to change drinking behaviour

Table 18.4 (*Continued*)

Action	Description

11. Screen for and treat any identified psychiatric problem	• Depression: usually remits within a few weeks of abstinence; if it persists beyond 3–4 weeks of abstinence from alcohol, consider SSRI but be aware they may exacerbate the tremor, anxiety and insomnia common in people recently detoxified and they are more effective if used alongside therapy for the alcohol use disorder. There is an association between alcohol use disorders and suicide, so monitor suicide risk closely
	• Anxiety and insomnia: may persist for months post detox and may contribute to early relapse. Consider treatment if persist for more than 3–4 weeks after abstinence:
	  – Benzodiazepines may suppress but impaired psychomotor skills, risk of dependence and overdose (more likely to be lethal if in combination with alcohol), dependence on alcohol and benzodiazepines are associated with an increase in depressive symptoms and may be harder to treat than alcohol dependence alone; diazepam, lorazepam and alprazolam have greater abuse potential than chlordiazepoxide and oxazepam
	  – Buspirone: is less sedating than benzodiazepines, does not interact with alcohol to impair psychomotor skills, does not have abuse potential, can reduce anxiety in anxious dependent people with people who have high baseline anxiety scores doing better, but is no more effective than placebo in anxious severely alcohol-dependent people
	• Social phobia: untreated may perpetuate alcohol use disorders
	Treat with cognitive behavioural therapy with or without SSRI

12. ADHD	• Untreated may hinder treatment of alcohol use disorder • Psychostimulants can be safe and effective but have potential for abuse, and ongoing alcohol use can limit their efficacy • Start treatment with non-stimulant medication, but consider stimulant if an adequate response is not obtained • Base decision to start stimulant medication on multidisciplinary team assessment and risk–benefit analysis and discontinue if alcohol use worsens or if evidence of diversion of prescribed medications • Consider slow-release stimulant medication, as may have less abuse potential
13. Co-morbid substance misuse	• Smoking: encourage to stop smoking and refer to local stop smoking supports • Co-morbid opioid use: treat both conditions actively and be aware of increased mortality with taking opioids and alcohol together • Co-morbid stimulant, cannabis or benzodiazepine use: treat both conditions actively. In alcohol withdrawal regime using benzodiazepine, it is good practice to convert to one benzodiazepine, for example, diazepam, and increase the dose for the withdrawal tapering over 2–3 weeks back to the original dose and then slowly reduce the diazepam dose over time

Source: Data from Mendel and Hipkins (2002).

MODERATE TO SEVERE WITHDRAWAL IN ADULTS WITH ID IS COMPLICATED BY:

- Communication problems
- Obtaining accurate information about the amount and pattern of drinking and current and past withdrawal reactions
- Frequency of physical and psychiatric co-morbidities
- Lack of adapted questionnaires and measurement tools
- Impairment in the capacity to consent to treatment

    It is therefore recommended that in this group the multidisciplinary team is involved in planning for the detox and that specialist addictions service input is sought. The local ID service may wish to support their service users to receive detoxes on local addictions wards rather than attempt the detox on ID inpatient units, which have less experience in alcohol detoxes. Inpatient admissions should be for 2–3 weeks, minimum.

Illustrative case study 18.3

Joe is 22, has ADHD and mild ID and presents after the police bring him to hospital. The police had been called because Joe was shouting obscenities at females in the street, and when they approached him, he became very disturbed and aggressive. At interview, he reports drinking heavily since his psychostimulant medication was stopped when he was 18. He has multiple convictions for shoplifting alcohol and for violence associated offences. At interview, he reports that his ex-girlfriend is telling him to shout at women and is interfering with his thoughts and controlling him. He is diagnosed with paranoid schizophrenia and transferred to a secure hospital under the Mental Health Act where he receives treatment for his alcohol dependence (individual and motivational therapy) and for schizophrenia. He is transferred back to an open ward on antipsychotic depot and oral naltrexone, and a supported community placement is sought.

Discussion case study 18.4

A 56-year-old lady with mild ID is brought to the attention of the local ID services by her adult son. She has been drinking heavily for many years and despite multiple inpatient detoxes has never remained abstinent for more than a few months or fully engaged in treatment. She has experienced withdrawal seizures in the past and has also been admitted to hospital following head injuries sustained in domestic violence on many occasions. She has always said she wants to continue to drink. Her son reports a gradual increase in forgetfulness and deterioration in her self-care and care of her house. She has also lost weight.

- What are the diagnostic possibilities?
- What management strategies could be tried?
- What is the role of medication in this case?

Medication is also used to control drinking, either by producing unpleasant effects when alcohol is consumed or by moderating the neurotransmitter systems that medicate alcohol reinforcement.

Table 18.5 describes the evidence base for medication treatment in alcohol use disorders, and Table 18.6 outlines a possible reducing regime for treatment of alcohol withdrawal.

Table 18.5 Role of medication treatments in alcohol use disorders.

Medication	Use and evidence
Medication treatments of alcohol withdrawal	
1. Benzodiazepines: suppress the hyperexcitability of alcohol withdrawal by acting as GABA agonists	• Diazepam and chlordiazepoxide are used most commonly in reducing regimes because they are long acting and effectively self-tapering. They are metabolised through the liver • National Institute for Health and Care Excellence (2010, 2011) recommend fixed or symptom-triggered protocols for assisted withdrawal • In impaired liver function, oxazepam or lorazepam may be considered as they are not metabolised to long-acting metabolites and carry less risk of accumulation
2. Antiepileptics	• Carbamazepine has been found to be equal to lorazepam in its ability to reduce symptoms of alcohol withdrawal and to be particularly useful in people with multiple episodes of withdrawal. NICE Guidance (National Institute for Health and Care Excellence, 2010, 2011) recommends offering either benzodiazepines or carbamazepine to treat symptoms of acute alcohol withdrawal • Valproate has been found to be useful as an adjunct when prescribed with benzodiazepines • Gabapentin has shown no advantage over placebo • Carbamazepine and valproate are metabolised through the liver, and valproate may increase the risk of hepatotoxicity, so, given liver function may be impaired in alcohol use disorders, it is important to monitor carefully both liver function and medication blood levels when using these medications
3. Chlormethiazole	• May be offered as alternative to benzodiazepine or carbamazepine but should be used with caution, in inpatient settings only and according to the summary of product characteristics (National Institute for Health and Care Excellence, 2010)
Medication treatments to control drinking **1. Alcohol-sensitising agents** • Disulfiram (Antabuse) inhibits the enzyme ALDH that catalyses the oxidation of acetaldehyde to acetic acid. Drinking alcohol within two weeks of taking disulfiram causes the disulfiram–ethanol reaction (DER). The DER includes flushing, increased heart rate, decreased blood pressure, nausea, vomiting, shortness of breath, sweating, dizziness, blurred vision and confusion. It lasts about 30 minutes and is usually self-limiting but can be severe, and cardiovascular collapse and seizures are rare complications. The severity of the reaction varies with the dose of disulfiram and amount of alcohol taken	• Disulfiram: In controlled studies, there is no or minimal advantage over placebo. It may have some benefit in men who cannot remain abstinent. Users need to understand that they must avoid all alcohol even that in over-the-counter preparations, food and medications that interact with it. In general, its use would not be recommended in people with ID unless recommended by an addictions specialist and in the context of a risk–benefit analysis, capacity assessment and close working between the ID and addictions services

(Continued)

Table 18.5 (*Continued*)

Medication	Use and evidence
2. Medications to reduce the reinforcing effects of alcohol	
• Naltrexone: opioid antagonist • Acamprosate: amino acid derivative, which affects both GABA and excitatory amino acids such as glutamate • Antiepileptics • SSRIs	• Start treatment as soon as possible after assisted withdrawal • NICE recommends oral naltrexone or oral acamprosate • Naltrexone: – Advantages over placebo in promoting abstinence, preventing relapse to heavy drinking and reducing drinking days – Optimal length of treatment is 6 months, and then gradual increase in relapse rate occurs – It may be more effective when combined with CBT or supportive therapy – Long-acting oral and injectable preparations may improve benefit, and combining with acamprosate results in lower relapse rate (but note that the study is not fully randomised) – Start at 25 mg a day and aim for maintenance dose of 50 mg/day for 6 months or longer if benefitting – Stop if drinking persists for 4–6 weeks after starting the medication – Ensure service user is aware of its impact on opioid-based analgesics – Monitor monthly at clinic and advise service user that if they feel unwell they must immediately stop naltrexone • Acamprosate: – Beneficial in relapse prevention and has good safety profile – Usually prescribed at dose of 666 mg three times a day for 6 months or longer if benefitting – Stop if drinking persists for 4–6 weeks after starting the medication • Antiepileptics: there is evidence that carbamazepine, valproate and topiramate can be useful in treating alcohol dependence • SSRIs: fluoxetine and citalopram are the most heavily studied. The literature suggests they are only effective in people with earlier onset of and less severe dependency

Table 18.6 A reducing regime for treatment of alcohol withdrawal.

Fixed-dose regime (assess severity of dependence before starting regime and alter regime accordingly; for use in community and inpatient settings)

Day	Dose of chlordiazepoxide
1	25 mg four times a day
2	20 mg four times a day
3	15 mg four times a day
4	10 mg four times a day
5	10 mg three times a day
6	5 mg three times a day
7	5 mg twice a day
8	5 mg at night

Symptom-triggered dosing regimes (for use in inpatient settings only)

Symptom-triggered regimes	Example of a symptom-triggered regime
Use where people with acute alcohol withdrawal are in settings where 24 hour assessment and monitoring are available (such as inpatient units) and where staff are competent in monitoring symptoms effectively and the unit has sufficient resources to allow them to do so frequently and safely. ID inpatient unit staff may not have the right training and experience to be able to follow symptom-triggered regimes	On days 1–4, chlordiazepoxide 20–30 mg as needed up to hourly, based on symptoms (including pulse rate greater than 90 per minute, diastolic pressure greater than 90 mmHg or signs of withdrawal)

Source: Data from National Institute for Health and Care Excellence (2010).

References

Cooper SA, Smiley E, Morison J, Williamson A, Allan A. (2007) Mental ill-health in adults with intellectual disability. *British Journal of Psychiatry* 190:27–35.

Mendel E, Hipkins J. (2002) Motivating learning disabled offenders with alcohol-related problems: a pilot study. *British Journal of Learning Disabilities* 30(4):153–158.

Taggart L, McLaughlin D, Quinn B, Milligan V. (2006) An exploration of substance misuse in people with intellectual disabilities. *Journal of Intellectual Disability Research* 50(8):588–597.

Further reading

Alcohol Concern. (n.d.) Available at http://www.alcoholconcern.org.uk (accessed 8 January 2015).

BILD. (n.d.) *Alcohol and smoking, illustrated booklet.* Available at http://www.bild.org.uk/our-services/books/health-and-wellbeing/alcohol-and-smoking (accessed 8 January 2015).

Kranzier H, Ciraulo D. (2005) Alcohol. In: Kranzler H, Ciraulo D, eds. *Clinical manual of addictions psychopharmacology.* American Psychiatric Publishing, Washington, DC, pp. 1–545.

Levin R. (2007) ADHD and substance abuse update. *American Journal on Addictions* 16:1–4.

Mariani J, Levin F. (2007) Treatment strategies for co-occurring ADHD and substance use disorders. *American Journal on Addictions* 16:45–56.

Miller H, Whicher E. (2009) Substance misuse. In: Hassiotis A, Barron A, Hall I, eds. *Intellectual disability psychiatry: a practical handbook*. John Wiley & Sons, Inc., Hoboken, NJ.

National Institute for Health and Care Excellence. (2010) Alcohol-use disorders: diagnosis and clinical management of alcohol-related physical complications. NICE guidelines CG100. Available at www.nice.org.uk/guidance/CG100 (accessed 8 January 2015).

National Institute for Health and Care Excellence. (2011) Alcohol-use disorders: diagnosis, assessment and management of harmful drinking and alcohol dependence. NICE guidelines CG115. Available at www.nice.org.uk/guidance/CG115 (accessed 8 January 2015).

National Institute for Health and Care Excellence. (2010) Alcohol-use disorders: sample chlordiazepoxide dosing regimes for use in managing alcohol withdrawal. Available at http://www.nice.org.uk/nicemedia/live/13337/53105/53105.pdf (accessed 16 February 2015).

CHAPTER 19

Personality Disorders

Regi Alexander[1] & Sabyasachi Bhaumik[2,3]

[1]*Partnerships in Care, Norfolk & Norwich Medical School, University of East Anglia, Norfolk, UK*
[2]*Leicestershire Partnership NHS Trust, Leicester, UK*
[3]*Department of Health Sciences, University of Leicester, Leicester, UK*

> Living with Borderline Personality Disorder is one hell of a ride. It's hard, it's scary, it's passionate, it's angry and it's everything in between.
>
> *borderlinelife.tumblr.com/*

Definition

Personality disorders, whether defined using ICD-10 or DSM-IV, would broadly fall within three major clusters: flamboyant (which includes borderline, antisocial, histrionic and narcissistic), eccentric (which includes paranoid, schizoid and schizotypal) and the anxious/fearful (which includes obsessive compulsive, avoidant and dependent behaviours).

Key points specific to intellectual disability

The diagnosis of personality disorder in those with intellectual disability (ID) can be a contentious issue. Difficulties in eliciting the information necessary for the diagnosis due to communication difficulties; the overlap between characteristics of either the person's ID or other developmental disabilities, such as autism spectrum disorders with some of the personality disorder criteria; the lack of valid and reliable instruments; the differences in the criteria adopted by various classificatory systems; and the overlap of transient psychotic and affective symptoms in both psychiatric illnesses, as well as some personality disorders, all contribute to this. The variability in prevalence figures together with issues around diagnostic

---

The Frith Prescribing Guidelines for People with Intellectual Disability, Third Edition.
Edited by Sabyasachi Bhaumik, David Branford, Mary Barrett and Satheesh Kumar Gangadharan.
© 2015 John Wiley & Sons, Ltd. Published 2015 by John Wiley & Sons, Ltd.

reliability and validity have been extensively reviewed and commented on. Whatever the controversies, the personality disorder diagnosis still appears to be clinically relevant because it may affect a person's acceptance into community placements, predict subsequent psychiatric disorders, determine the rate of referral to specialist services, influence the mode of treatment and affect long-term treatment outcomes. Due to the difficulties in making this diagnosis in those with severe degrees of disability, there appears to be a general consensus that it should, at present, be limited to those within the mild and moderate ranges of ID. Adopting these parameters, it appears that the prevalence figure for the diagnosis within those who are in contact with community services for ID would be around 7% and for those within forensic services around 49–59%.

Medication treatments for personality disorders in general psychiatry

Although no medication has been licensed specifically for the treatment of personality disorders, they are much used in clinical practice.

Definition

Personality disorders, whether defined using ICD-10 or DSM-IV, would broadly fall within three major clusters: flamboyant (which includes borderline, antisocial, histrionic and narcissistic), eccentric (which includes paranoid, schizoid and schizotypal) and the anxious/fearful (which includes obsessive compulsive, avoidant and dependent behaviours).

To clearly establish the efficacy of any treatment in personality disorder, four strict conditions would need to be satisfied. These include:

1 The treatment should be effective in the pure form of the personality disorder (i.e. independent of co-morbidity).
2 Efficacy should be established using the methodology of the randomised controlled trial (RCT) (despite the inherent difficulties of using this methodology for personality disorders).
3 Because there are no established medication treatments, any treatment tested has to be superior in efficacy to placebo, using the methodology described above.
4 Treatment should show evidence of efficacy over a period of at least 6 months in view of the long duration of personality disorder.

It would be fair to say that none of the current medication treatments would satisfy all of the above criteria. However, the disruption and distress caused by people with personality disorder (both to themselves and others) is such that, more often than not, treatment with psychotropic medications occurs at some point in their psychiatric history. The conventional approach to medication treatment in the field of mental health is the one based on clinical diagnosis. This works well, particularly if the syndrome being treated is a clear-cut psychiatric illness. A second approach would be a 'symptom-based' one. This has been favoured in the field of personality disorders, and the reasons for it have been well elucidated.

General adult psychiatry: Medication treatments based on the personality disorder diagnosis

Flamboyant cluster: Borderline personality disorder

Two early placebo-controlled RCTs using low-dose haloperidol and low-dose thiothixene showed the effectiveness of these medications in reducing typical borderline behaviour and associated symptoms including depression; however, the results of subsequent studies have been equivocal. Improvements do not seem to last beyond 16 weeks, and there is a problem with poor compliance and adverse effects even on small doses. There is RCT evidence that olanzapine is superior to placebo for borderline symptoms, except depression, and that it was superior to placebo for global improvement in borderline personality. One RCT shows superiority for fluoxetine over placebo in reducing anger, and another RCT showed that selective serotonin reuptake inhibitors (SSRIs) reduced impulsiveness and deliberate self-harm. Studies comparing tricyclics, mainly amitriptyline, with placebo or other medications have given different results, which make interpretation difficult and lead to the suggestion that more than one type of borderline personality disorder exists, with different types responding to different therapies. Monoamine oxidase inhibitors (MAOIs) like phenelzine and tranylcypromine may be effective.

Flamboyant cluster: Antisocial personality disorder

Based on anecdotal reports, low-dose antipsychotics, including depot preparations, have been recommended for many years. Two studies from the 1970s showed lithium to reduce anger and impulsiveness in this group of people, but the findings have not been replicated.

Odd, eccentric cluster

Very little evidence is available on the effectiveness of antipsychotics or other psychotropic medications in the treatment of this group.

Anxious, fearful cluster

There is difficulty in interpreting data from these personality disorders because a mood state – anxiety – predominates in this group and the beneficial effects of medications may well be a consequence of their effects on mood rather than personality. There is also a problem of diagnostic overlap: the one between anxious (avoidant) personality disorder and social phobia being most prominent. Antidepressants in general seem to have some value in treatment and are widely used. Benzodiazepines have also been used.

General adult psychiatry: Medication treatments based on the personality disorder predominant symptom domain

The rationale for the symptom domain-based approach to medication treatment in personality disorders has been well elucidated. Much of the core theoretical foundations for this approach stem from the temperament–character–intelligence (TCI) model of personality advocated by Cloninger et al. (1993). This approach has been reflected in the most recent guidelines from the American Psychiatric Association (APA) on the treatment of borderline personality disorder. The target symptom domains of personality disorders identified in this manner are:
• Behaviour dyscontrol, which includes affective aggression, predatory aggression, organic-like aggression and ictal aggression
• Mood dysregulation, which includes emotional lability and depression/anxiety/ psychotic symptoms
Medications of choice as well as contraindicated medications for each of these domains have been proposed.

Psychiatry of ID: Issues in the diagnosis and treatment of personality disorders

Published literature on medication treatments in this area is very limited and mostly limited to case series or small retrospective surveys. One case series reported on 20 mentally retarded offenders with personality disorders. The treatment package included, among other things, medication therapy in 70% of people. Medications used included tranquillisers, sex suppressants, hypnotics, anxiolytics and antidepressants. Further details are not mentioned; however, overall, the treatment programme had a good or fair response in 85% of cases. Another report described two cases, one with paranoid personality disorder and the other with an obsessive personality disorder. Medication treatment was a part of the comprehensive treatment package and included a low-dose antipsychotic medication (details not given) for the former and an SSRI (fluvoxamine) for the latter. The overall treatment response appeared favourable. In a series of three cases of borderline personality disorder, olanzapine was used in two cases and a fluoxetine–divalproex sodium combination in the other. Medication treatment was combined with psychotherapy or behavioural strategies. A four-stage model for the management of borderline personality disorder has been proposed (Wilson, 2001); this author reported a case study illustrating the effective implementation of the model in a 48-year-old woman. Medication treatment in this case included venlafaxine, trazodone, carbamazepine, risperidone and lorazepam. A retrospective study on the use of clozapine in ID described three people with a personality disorder who were treated beneficially with the medication. There have been a number of studies giving accounts of the use of clozapine in various kinds of behavioural problems (including aggression and self-injury) in ID; further details of these can be found in the reference list at the end of this chapter. In an audit on the pharmacotherapy of personality disorder in an outpatient sample of patients with ID, the main symptom domains for treatment were explored. Cognitive perceptual (psychosis-like) symptoms were present in 48%; symptoms of affective dysregulation in 79%; symptoms of behaviour dyscontrol, impulsivity and aggression in 97%; symptoms of anxiety in 34%; and self-injurious behaviour in 52%. As expected, most people had features from two or more domains: all five symptom domains being present in 3 (10%), four domains in 10 (34%), three domains in 6 (21%) and two domains in 5 (17%). The flow chart for the medication treatment of personality disorders in ID follows the 'targeting of a predominant symptom domain' approach. In that sense, it is an adaptation of the similar approach in general psychiatry. The different domains that are proposed here are self-evident, not mutually exclusive, and there is bound to be a considerable degree of overlap between them. It therefore follows that for the same person, the clinician may need to apply different stems of this flow chart. The view about the medication treatment of personality disorders remaining 'a clouded area governed more by opinion than fact' seems to have even more of a ring of truth when it comes to ID. Notwithstanding all these limitations, this chapter is a preliminary effort to examine within a structured and systematic theoretical framework the use of psychotropic medications in this population. Perhaps we should console ourselves that Tyrer stated in 1998 that 'the current medication treatment of personality disorder is like following a badly marked track through a dense fog – seeing only a short distance ahead, but grateful for any guidance going' (Tyrer, 1998). The following audit standards have been suggested for monitoring psychotropic medication use in this group:

1 The person's multiaxial diagnosis should be recorded in the case notes.
2 Pharmacological treatment should only be part of a multidisciplinary treatment package.
3 The predominant symptom complex(es) being targeted for medication treatment should be recorded.
4 Expected improvements and behavioural targets should be identified in discussion with the person and recorded before the start of treatment.
5 Discussions about the rationale, effects and potential side effects of the proposed treatment with the person and, if appropriate, with his carer/advocate should be recorded.
6 There should be regular follow-up appointments to monitor progress on these expected changes. A clear record of any symptomatic improvement, worsening or side effects should be kept during this follow-up.
7 There should be an agreement on the length of time that the person will be tried on a medication. If there are no beneficial effects within that time, the medication should be stopped.

Illustrative case study 19.1

Elizabeth is a 30-year-old lady with a mild ID and a long history of behavioural problems including aggression towards people and property, threats and acts of self-harm and repeated inappropriate attendance at A&E departments. From late childhood, she experienced sexual abuse by her father and felt abandoned by her mother. From her teenage years, she was caught up in a series of abusive relationships with older men. She used to have significant mood swings – periods of well-being and excessive cheerfulness interspersed with periods of extreme irritability and low mood – this could happen several times in the same week. At times of stress, this could happen in the same day and be accompanied by aggressive acting out or self-harming. She had a very ambiguous relationship with the community ID team – at times describing them as her only hope and at other times blaming them for trying to control her life or not offering her enough help. This would be accompanied by threats to self-harm or harm others. She would occasionally talk about 'hearing voices' when stressed. A detailed diagnostic clarification suggested the presence of an emotionally unstable personality disorder. The affective symptoms did not reach the threshold for the diagnosis of a major mood disorder, nor was there evidence to support a diagnosis of a psychotic illness. Since features of affective dysregulation were most prominent, she was treated with sodium valproate within BNF limits as a mood stabiliser. This was in addition to her attending mindfulness sessions and therapy through the psychology department.

Note 1: Many authors suggest that the use of multiple treatment modalities – pharmacological and psychological – would provide increased benefit in terms of treatment outcome.

Note 2: The predominant symptom domains adapted for use in personality disorders in ID are:

- Behaviour dyscontrol/aggression/impulsivity:
  - Affective aggression: impulsive, hot tempered, associated with mood changes, often normal EEGs
  - Predatory aggression: hostility and cruel
  - Organic-like aggression
  - Ictal aggression: often associated with epilepsy/abnormal EEGs
- Mood dysregulation:
  - Mood swings or mood instability
  - Dysthymia-like symptoms or emotional detachment
- Anxiety symptoms:
  - Predominant cognitive anxiety
  - Predominant somatic anxiety
- 'Psychotic' symptoms:
  - Chronic low-level symptoms
  - Acute symptoms/acts of deliberate self-harm

Note 3: Although there are more studies on the use of lithium, there may be practical difficulties with blood tests, monitoring, etc. Therefore, medications like carbamazepine or valproate may need to be used instead.

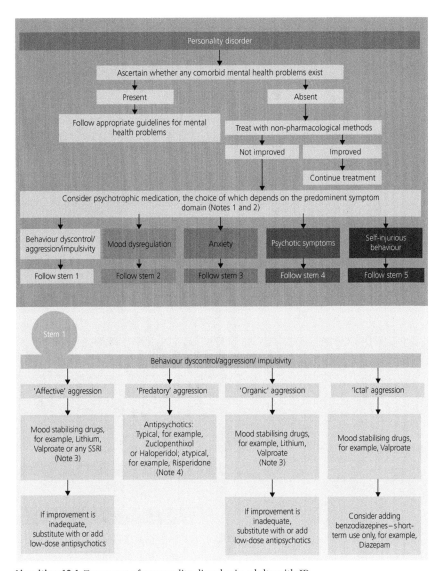

Algorithm 19.1 Treatment of personality disorder in adults with ID.

Note 4: There is inadequate data to recommend a specific antipsychotic medication. Although there is some RCT evidence for the usefulness of zuclopenthixol tablets, many clinicians may prefer an atypical antipsychotic because of the better side effect profile.

Note 5: The use of opiate antagonists like naltrexone has been reviewed in the guidelines from the APA on the management of deliberate self-harm in borderline personality disorder.

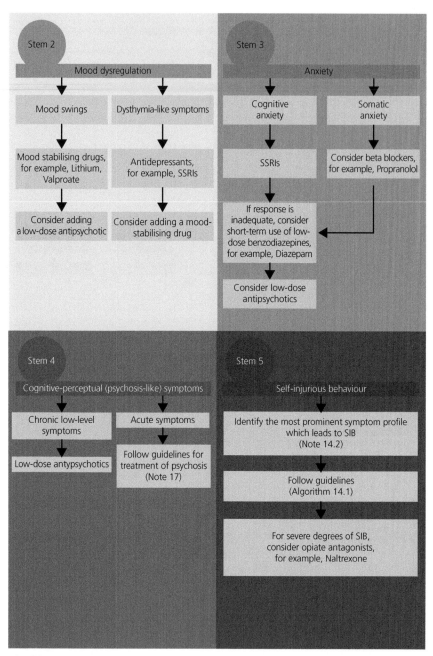

Algorithm 19.1 (*Continued*)

Discussion case study 19.2

> James is a 26-year-old Caucasian male with a mild level of intellectual disability. His problems started from late childhood; although ADHD was queried, a definitive diagnosis was not made. As a young adult, his behavioural problems included severe aggression towards people and property. He had very poor frustration tolerance and would act out without thinking, blame others for his actions, abuse alcohol and illicit medications and steal or indulge in similar antisocial behaviours. He had a number of girlfriends, often people who were less able than him, and he was prone to be violent towards them after arguments. He would report hearing voices at times, when he was stressed. These would last for up to a week or 2 weeks during which time, he would be very disturbed and neglecting his personal care.
> - What is the differential diagnosis?
> - Which symptoms should be initially targeted for treatment?
> - What is your medication group of choice?
> - How should medication treatment be titrated to best manage James's condition?

References

Cloninger CR, Svrakic DM, Przybeck TR (1993) A psychobiological model of temperament and character. *Arch Gen Psychiatry* 50: 975–90.

Tyrer P (1998) Medication treatment of personality disorder. *Psychiatr Bull* 22(4): 242–4.

Wilson SR (2001) A four-stage model for management of borderline personality disorder in people with mental retardation. *Ment Health Aspects Dev Disabil* 4: 68–76.

Further reading

Alexander R, Cooray S (2003) Diagnosis of personality disorders in learning disability. *Br J Psychiatry* 182(44): 28–31.

Alexander RT, Crouch K, Halstead S, Piachaud J (2006) Long term outcome from a medium secure service for people with intellectual disability. *J Intellect Disabil Res* 49(4): 305–15.

Alexander R, Tajuddin M, Gangadharan SK (2007) Personality disorders in intellectual disability – approaches to pharmacotherapy. *Ment Health Aspects Dev Disabil* 10(4): 129–36.

Biswas AB, Gibbons S, Gangadharan S (2006) Clozapine in borderline personality disorder and intellectual disability: a case report of four-year outcome. *Ment Health Aspects Dev Disabil* 9(1): 13–17.

Bogenshutz MP, Nurnberg HG (2001) Olanzapine versus placebo in the treatment of borderline personality disorder. *J Clin Psychiatry* 64: 104–9.

Goldberg SC, Shulz SC, Schulz PM, Resnick RJ, Hamer RM, Friedel RO (1986) Borderline and schizotypal personality disorders treated with low dose thiothixine versus placebo. *Arch Gen Psychiatry* 43: 680–6.

Hammock RG, Schroeder SR, Levine WR (1995) The effect of clozapine on self-injurious behaviour. *J Autism Dev Disord* 25: 611–26.

Hammock R, Levine WR, Schroeder SR (2001) Brief report: effects of clozapine on self-injurious behaviour of two risperidone nonresponders with mental retardation. *J Autism Dev Disord* 31: 109–13.

Kingston NY, Mavromatis M (2000) The diagnosis and treatment of borderline personality disorder in persons with developmental disability – 3 case reports. *Ment Health Aspects Dev Disabil* 3: 89–97.

Lindsay WR, Gabriel S, Dana L, Young S, Dosen A (2005) Personality disorders. In: Fletcher R, Loschen E, Sturmey P, eds. *Diagnostic Manual of Psychiatric Disorders for Individuals with Mental Retardation*. National Association for Dual Diagnosis, Kingston, NY.

Naik BI, Gangadharan SK, Alexander RT (2002) Personality disorders in learning disability – the clinical experience. *Br J Dev Disabil* 48: 95–100.

Oldham JM (2005) *Guideline Watch: Practice Guideline for the Treatment of Patients with Borderline Personality Disorder*. American Psychiatric Association, Arlington, VA. Available at: http://psychiatryonline.org/pb/assets/raw/sitewide/practice_guidelines/guidelines/bpd-watch.pdf (accessed 26 February 2015).

Salzman C, Woolfson AN, Schatzberg A, et al. (1995) Effect of fluoxetine on anger in symptomatic volunteers with borderline personality disorder. *J Clin Psychopharmacol* 15: 23–9.

Thalayasingam S, Alexander RT, Singh I (2004) The use of clozapine in adults with intellectual disability. *J Intellect Disabil Res* 48(Pt 6): 572–9.

Tyrer P (2001) *Personality Disorders – Diagnosis, Management and Course*. 2nd edn. Butterworth Heinemann, Oxford.

Verkes RJ, Van der Mast RC, Kerkhof AJ, et al. (1998) Platelet serotonin, monoamine oxidase activity, and [3H]paroxetine binding related to impulsive suicide attempts and borderline personality disorder. *Biol Psychiatry* 43: 740–6.

Zanarini MC, Frankenburg FR (2001) Olanzapine treatment of female borderline personality disorder patients: a double blind, placebo-controlled pilot study. *J Clin Psychiatry* 61: 849–53.

CHAPTER 20

Discussion Case Studies with Suggested Answers

Epilepsy

A 44-year-old lady with autism and generalised epilepsy who lives in a supported living accommodation is seen in your clinic for a review of her epilepsy control. You notice that over the past two years, her lamotrigine has been gradually increased by your trainee doctors to a maximum of 125 mg twice daily with no success in controlling her tonic–clonic seizures.

On further history taking, you realise that she self-administers her medication but has not let her support workers in to monitor the administration of medication. Further observation by the staff, who finally manage to get into her flat, reveals that she has hoarded her medication over the past 12 months. You arrange for another review but notice that she becomes extremely anxious when you discuss compliance with treatment. She also appears confused when you discuss side effects and struggles to repeat what you have just explained to her in spite of appearing fluent superficially.

- **What are the main issues in the management of her epilepsy?**
  It seems that compliance is the main issue in this scenario. Although she appears able and verbally fluent on the surface, it may be that she struggles with comprehending the information given to her about the risks of untreated epilepsy and beneficial as well as the side effects of antiepileptic medication.
- **What are the risks in this case?**
  Risks include SUDEP and injuries from uncontrolled seizures especially because she is living alone. It is therefore paramount to involve the multidisciplinary team including a social worker.
- **Who else would you involve in your management plan?**
  Help from a speech and language therapist (SLT) in providing accessible information on epilepsy would be paramount in her management plan.

The Frith Prescribing Guidelines for People with Intellectual Disability, Third Edition.
Edited by Sabyasachi Bhaumik, David Branford, Mary Barrett and Satheesh Kumar Gangadharan.
© 2015 John Wiley & Sons, Ltd. Published 2015 by John Wiley & Sons, Ltd.

This is extremely important in engaging her in the treatment plan. A community nurse can also help to build up a therapeutic relationship with her, which as a result might improve her compliance. The social worker can provide input by commissioning twice daily calls for home support and supervising administration of her lamotrigine. Environmental adaptations by the colleagues from the occupational therapy team are also important (see the following).

- **What are the non-pharmacological aspects of treating her epilepsy?**
  Environmental adaptations such as setting up an epilepsy bed sensor along with other assistive technologies facilitating access to her flat during out-of-hours period by the staff and emergency team would ensure that risk of SUDEP and injuries are minimised. These and other strategies could be incorporated in detail in her epilepsy care plan/health action plan.

Dementia

Brenda is a 55-year-old lady with Down syndrome living in a residential home. Carers report deterioration in her personal hygiene, which they attribute to loss of personal care skills. She tends to lose her way around the home. She is often forgetful and accuses other residents of stealing her things. According to care staff, these changes have been noted since the demise of her mother 6 months ago, at which point she came to live at this home. She has poor sleep at night and has been found by carers on occasions in the back garden appearing confused. She has mild ID and was not previously known to services. She has now been referred by the GP for further assessment.

- **How will you assess this case?**
  Assessment should follow the nine-step approach described by the National Task Group on Intellectual Disabilities and Dementia Practices (Mayo Clinic Proceedings 2013). This is discussed in detail in the chapter in Table 5.3 and Algorithm 5.1 and please refer to the same for full description of the pathway to follow. Key points to remember here would be communication difficulties that could preclude history taking, pre-existing cognitive impairment due to Down syndrome, presence of sensory impairment and autism and difficulties with medical investigations.

- **What are the diagnostic possibilities?**
  It is important to rule out conditions that mimic dementia before a diagnosis of dementia is made as many conditions cause reversible cognitive impairment and if identified correctly can be treated.
  - Physical health problems – Hypothyroidism, anaemia, vitamin B_{12} or folate deficiencies, hypo- or hyperglycaemia, electrolyte disturbances, etc.
  - Other brain conditions – Haematoma, infections affecting the brain as well as brain tumours
  - Mental health conditions – Depression, psychotic conditions, severe forms of anxiety, etc.
  - Medications – Raised levels of antiepileptic medications, medications with anticholinergic side effects, multiple medications, etc.

- ○ Psychosocial – Bereavement, loss of contact with key individuals, changes in day activities, any significant stressful life events (e.g. sexual or physical abuse), etc.
- ○ Environment – Increased demand from a new environment and lack of adequate stimulation in the environment
- ○ Sensory impairments – Hearing deficits, visual impairment (cataract), etc.
- **What will be the management plan?**
  Management plan once a diagnosis of dementia is made
  For the management of cognitive symptoms, cholinesterase inhibitors are the mainstay of treatment. Please refer to Table 5.4 for full information on the use of AChE inhibitors in people with ID and dementia. Poor sleep and reversal of sleep–wake cycle are common in dementia and have to be managed using appropriate sleep hygiene measures and use of hypnotic medications (i.e. melatonin) if needed.

Eating and drinking

Adam is a 40-year-old man with ID and Down syndrome. He attends his annual health check at the GP surgery. The health check identifies that he is losing weight.
- **What is the GP role?**
- Review medication.
  - ○ Physical health check.
  - ○ Analyse re weight loss: If under 10% encourage regular meals and snacks, consider need for over the counter multivitamin/non-prescribable supplements. If over 10%, refer to dietetics for full nutritional assessment and advice. Analyse reasons for weight loss with carer.
  - ○ Enquire more about the nature of difficulties at mealtimes.
It is clear that Adam is struggling to eat a full meal and coughs on occasion when eating. The GP refers to the ID specialist health team.
What recommendations would you expect to be made by:
A The dietitian
B The ID health team
The dietitian recommends continuing Food First advice (fortification of foods and choosing high-calorie foods) and makes a request for the GP to prescribe oral nutritional supplements.
The Speech and language therapist (SLT) assesses and makes recommendations for texture modification of food and drink. The SLT liaises with the GP to prescribe the drink thickener that Adam prefers and suits his needs.
The occupational therapist provides recommendations regarding Adam's environment and Adam's preferences. The occupational therapist may recommend new eating and drinking equipment to support Adam to eat his meals.
The community nursing team support the GP with any physical health needs identified by the GP and may screen for dementia.

Sleep

A 35-year-old man with mild ID is urgently referred by his GP with a chief complaint of being suicidal and only managing 2–3 hours of sleep at night. The sleep difficulties have been going on for the last 6 months and began following relationship difficulties with the man's long-term partner, resulting in him having to leave home and move back in with his mother. He has begun feeling very low and threatened several times to take an overdose.

The GP prescribed the man prn diazepam three months ago, which he began using regularly to help him get off to sleep. On questioning, he also admits to intermittently using cannabis and alcohol to help him settle at night. Despite this, he is still suffering from insomnia and is now saying that he cannot go on like this any longer.

• **What type of sleep disorder is he suffering from?**
  He suffers from insomnia secondary to a severe depressive disorder.

• **What are the most likely maintaining factors for his insomnia?**
  His misuse of drugs and alcohol, regular use of benzodiazepine agents and ongoing relationship difficulties are maintaining factors for his insomnia and depressive symptoms including suicidal ideation.

• **How would you manage the situation? What are your priorities?**
  The priority should be given to risk assessment and if needs be admission to a mental health unit to treat this depressive episode safely while helping him, through MDT involvement, with his social situation as well as providing psychological input and advice on avoiding maladaptive coping strategies and adhering to sleep hygiene. If sleep difficulties persist despite these interventions and are impacting on his quality of life and wellbeing, then a short trial of a hypnotic drug may be indicated (See Algorithm 7.1).

Women's issues

Pamela is a 36-year-old woman with mild to moderate ID presenting with complex epilepsy and severe challenging behaviour (aggression towards others) who is living in a residential care home. Her seizures have been fairly well controlled for more than 10 years with current combination of sodium valproate 1 g twice daily and carbamazepine 600 mg twice daily. At present, she still has clusters of partial seizures, lasting up to 60 seconds, mainly occurring before her menstrual period.

Pamela attends her regular review with the local ID psychiatrist and complains of increasingly growing facial hair, which she finds very distressing and wants treated. Carers report that for a number of years, she has been low in mood, quite irritable, argumentative and aggressive towards staff around her menstrual period. Her BMI is 32, and BP is 140/90 mmHg. She is compliant with her medication.

- **What are the diagnostic possibilities?**
1 Polycystic ovary syndrome (PCOS)/clinical hyperandrogenism – she has features of hirsutism, being overweight and BMI 32. She has been on sodium valproate for her epilepsy treatment since a young age (increased prevalence of PCOS in women using valproate, Harden C and Hu X).
2 Premenstrual syndrome and/or catamenial epilepsy – she presents with episodic complex partial seizures and irritability, agitation, low mood and breast tenderness especially around her menstrual period.
3 Challenging behaviour may be related to environmental issues or presenting symptoms of PMS.
- **What management strategies could be tried?**
Management strategies should include education and raising staff awareness on PMS and catamenial epilepsy, monitoring her mood and menstrual period in diary, support for pain relief, relaxation exercises and also managing her challenging behaviour with behavioural management. A referral to the community team for weight management, healthy eating and active lifestyle could be tried.
- **What is the role of medication in this case?**
To consider reviewing medication treatment for epilepsy, particularly looking into the option of replacing valproate with an alternative newer antiepileptic medication. She is already on acetazolamide for catamenial epilepsy, but she still has short-lasting complex partial seizures episodically. Other options are to try intermittent clobazam 10 mg tid or titrated up an increase dose of her antiepileptic medication around her menstrual period.

For associated metabolic aberrations related to PCOS, appropriate treatment with antidiabetic medication, for example, metformin and statins, can be considered for high blood glucose and cholesterol (Bargiota and Diamanti-Kandarakis, 2012).

Sexual disorders

Richard is a 55-year-old man with mild ID and epilepsy who had been resident in a long-stay ID facility since his teens. He is an informal patient and was described as a 'model' resident on the ward, helpful to staff and visitors, with no behavioural concerns reported in that environment. Richard attends the on-site sheltered workshop daily where he earns a therapeutic wage. He likes to go into the local town independently where he will spend his wages on sweets and comics. During these trips, he has repeatedly approached young adolescent boys and offered them sweets and comics in exchange for becoming his friend. On a number of these occasions, he has been reported to the police and charges brought; however, he has never been successfully prosecuted. Whenever there is an impending court appearance, Richard acknowledges his behaviour and appears keen to engage in treatment, but afterwards, he quickly disengages. Richard now has a reputation in the local community for this behaviour and has been physically assaulted on three separate occasions as a consequence. He however remains insistent on continuing his usual outings unaccompanied.

- **What are the risks?**

  Richard is at risk of further violence and aggression from others in the local community, and he does not appear to either acknowledge this risk; alternatively his drive to fulfil his wish to meet underage boys is stronger than his need to remain safe. Given his ID and behaviour pattern, he is therefore a vulnerable adult, as well as putting others at risk.

  Richard's pattern of behaviour and repeated unwillingness to engage in treatment makes it extremely unlikely his risk level will change in the near future.

- **How would you manage this situation?**

  Richard's clinical team looked at whether the Mental Health Act was applicable here, but it was not deemed that he was detainable. The role of the Mental Capacity Act was also considered: assessment highlighted that Richard had the capacity to make decisions in this matter and was aware of the potential consequences of his actions, albeit attempts to get a conviction in court have been unsuccessful to date. Given the potential risks highlighted earlier, however, the clinical team needed to engage with a number of agencies to manage that risk as best as practicable.

- **Which agencies should be involved and what is their role?**

  In addition to the ID service, key players here are social care and the police, with multi-agency working essential. The area police force has a specialist team who work with vulnerable adults, who were able to engage with Richard and have further dialogue with him around his behaviour and the resulting risk to both himself and others. This team then liaised with the local area police team to make them aware of the issues. A multi-agency meeting was held, and a management plan drawn up that the ID facility would alert the police on Richard leaving the facility, and the police would then check on his whereabouts. This acted as a deterrent to both the local population who were targeting him and to Richard in his attempts to engage with underage boys. The staff from the ID facility continued to work with Richard and to offer him support in the community to engage in appropriate activities away from risky situations, which he gradually became more accepting of over time.

ASD

Brian, a 72-year-old man with mild ID and ASD living in residential care becomes increasingly reluctant to go out of the house and participate in his usual day-care programme. He insists on spending increasing periods of time in his room arranging his collection of newspapers and magazines and becomes very agitated if the staff attempt to engage with him during this process. Over a period of weeks, he becomes increasingly nocturnal, not going to sleep until 3–4 AM, then staying in bed all morning. At this point, Brian is referred by his social worker to the community ID team for assessment and input.

- **What are the diagnostic possibilities?**

  The man's change in behaviour could indicate a number of possibilities. Physical health issues need to be explored, for example, deterioration in hearing and/or vision, hypothyroidism and other physical conditions; mental health causations could include depression, dementia, anxiety, OCD or even psychosis; environmental factors must be considered, for example, changes in staff, facilities or transport to the day centre can cause significant anxiety, also sensory factors such as a dislike of lighting or noise in certain environments; lastly, do not forget about possibilities such as abuse. Sometimes, it is not possible to identify the trigger for a change in behaviour at the time it occurs, but once occurred, the behaviour may self-perpetuate, without intervention.

- **What management strategies could be tried?**
A thorough assessment of all the areas listed earlier is indicated, with diagnosis and treatment according to condition. Functional analysis of the behaviour can be helpful in identifying triggers and possible management strategies. Prioritisation of symptoms for treatment is important: it is likely that key targets will be normalising his sleep pattern and reducing anxiety levels which should, in turn, reduce his obsessional behaviours.

- **What is the role of medication in this case?**
Sleep: Behavioural intervention and sleep hygiene measures to shift the sleep pattern should be tried in the first instance. A course of Melatonin may be helpful alongside this, with the timing of treatment gradually brought forward in line with the behavioural measures.

   Anxiety: Anxiety management and use of strategies such as swings and trampolines may be of significant benefit for anxiety reduction and should not be discounted because of Brian's age. Use of an SSRI may be extremely helpful, benefitting both anxiety levels and also improving sleep if this disturbance is related to anxiety. Risperidone may also be considered if symptoms warrant this and SSRI treatment is unsuccessful, although the clinician must be mindful of the potential health risks associated with this strategy and regularly review the need to continue treatment.

ADHD

Clare is 19 and has a moderate learning disability and ADHD. She was diagnosed with ADHD at age 11 and had been taking a slow-release preparation of methylphenidate for several years. The dose had been increased 6 months earlier following deterioration in her behaviour during the transition from home to supported living.

Clare's carers asked for an early review because Clare seemed to be rather low in mood and was losing weight and her sleep had deteriorated.

- **What do you need to consider during the appointment?**
Clare will need a full review of her physical and mental health at this point. It will be important to look at the reasons for her move into supported living and her understanding of the transition process and whether the placement is meeting her needs. You will also need to explore her emotional needs regarding contact with her previous home and family, school and activities as she may have had multiple changes in her life, some of which may be significant losses.

The timing and the detail around the deterioration during the transition may be very helpful in understanding any triggers for the deterioration. Is there any clear evidence that this was indeed an increase in symptoms indicative of ADHD or was it an episode of distressed and difficult behaviour during a period of change in her life? It will also be helpful to determine whether she had any physical health problems during the period of deterioration, which may have led to her not receiving the correct dose of methylphenidate, that is, vomiting, or indeed if the dose was being given accurately during the transition phase. The impact of the increase in medication during the transition will also need to be assessed. It would be important to clarify the chronology of the onset of the low mood, weight loss and poor sleep.

- **Could this deterioration be secondary to her methylphenidate treatment?**

  The deterioration during the transition period and her recent low mood, weight loss and sleep disturbance may all be secondary to the methylphenidate. Reduction in appetite causing weight loss is a common side effect of methylphenidate. The appetite reduction usually lasts for the duration of the time the medication is effective in reducing the symptoms of ADHD. The person's appetite generally improves late afternoon or early evening, if the slow-release medication is given in with breakfast therefore clarifying when they are keen to eat will clarify if the weight loss is due to medication-induced appetite suppression. Low mood can occur early or later in the treatment of ADHD with stimulants or atomoxetine; therefore, it is essential to check mood subjectively and objectively at each appointment. Sleep disturbance is a common side effect seen with stimulant medication, and it usually causes sleep onset difficulties but may also cause shortened duration of sleep.

- **What would be the treatment options at this point?**

  The review of mental and physical health issues and psychological and environmental issues should clarify the treatment plan. One likely hypothesis is that the behavioural disturbance was due to the transition phase and the methylphenidate was increased unnecessarily. The increased medication has subsequently caused a range of side effects demonstrated by her low mood, weight loss and sleep disturbance. This would be managed by reducing the dose back to the previous level and then to reassess whether she improves. An alternative explanation may be that the stimulant medication was causing an insidious onset of low mood and depressive symptoms resulting in the distressed and disruptive behaviours during transition, which were then exacerbated by an increase in the methylphenidate dose. Again, the treatment plan would involve reduction of the medication and then a reassessment to consider whether to withdraw this medication and then, if ADHD medication is still required, to select an alternative medication to treat the ADHD symptoms.

  In summary, therefore, if symptoms of depression occur in the context of ADHD treatment, it is always advisable to reduce or withdraw the medication for ADHD and then to reassess the symptoms.

Aggression

Amy, a 48-year-old woman with moderate ID, is admitted to the local inpatient unit following a number of assaults on staff as well as other people with ID. She lives with her elderly mother and attends the day centre. The behaviour was first reported by the day centre; however, on further clarification, her mother revealed that the behaviour has been ongoing since Amy's dad died 18 months ago and her mother has many bruises on her arms. She, however, stated that her daughter never means to hurt her but that Amy has been getting 'very difficult' about her personal care.

On admission, Amy is found to be in a poorly kempt state. She refuses to be separated from a bag of torn up papers, which she brought in to hospital with her, and spends hours rearranging the papers in piles. Her communication consists mainly of repetitive phrases. She tends to sit alone and is clearly aversive to physical touch and loud noises.

- **What assessment would she need?**
  Detailed history including current functioning, biological symptoms, duration of symptoms, current mood state, triggers for aggression and risks to others and self; ABC/functional analysis of behaviour/observation in different settings; physical exam and investigation for organic causes including bloods; and information about mum's needs/health.
- **What are the diagnostic possibilities?**
  Physical cause, for example, hypo-/hyperthyroidism, normal bereavement reaction, pathological grief reaction, depression, psychosis, worries about mum, abuse, iatrogenic due to meds and behaviour disorder/learned behaviour.
- **What treatment options would you consider?**
  Psychological/behavioural strategies first line including CBT/anger management, adapted as needed.

  Medication is the last resort, and only to be used in conjunction with other strategies, and if warranted due to the risks. Need to consider impact of meds on other physical health conditions and potential for drug–drug interactions. Consider capacity to consent/follow best interest process if lacking capacity.
- **Is there a role for medication here?**
  See Table 12.1. If used, start low and go slow. Need to monitor closely during titration and regularly thereafter. Withdraw if ineffective and consider trial of alternative. No drug of choice; however, Risperidone is often used first line, given its profile as an atypical antipsychotic.

Self-injurious behaviours

Lisa is a 21-year-old Caucasian female with mild ID. She moved into residential care four years ago, after her parents had difficulties managing her behaviours. She currently is unable to access day activities outside the home due to challenging behaviour. Behaviours include aggression (biting others, hitting out at others, screaming, shouting) and self-injurious behaviours (SIB) (slapping face, head banging, biting wrists).

The staff report Lisa to be experiencing marked mood fluctuations and a disturbed sleep pattern. They have also noticed that Lisa's SIB increases after family visits and premenstrually. Lisa's placement is now at risk.

- **What are the diagnostic possibilities?**
  This could represent maladaptive learned behaviour, an adjustment reaction to change in circumstances, sociocultural issues (e.g. a reaction to changes in the residential home and abuse), communication difficulties causing Lisa frustration, a physical health disorder (e.g. dental pain, PMS, earache or constipation) and bipolar affective disorder (possibly rapid cycling).

- **What treatment strategies could be tried?**
  A thorough assessment involving physical and mental health factors is key to diagnosing those disorders. If present, they should be treated according to condition. A period of observation coupled with functional analysis will be required in the assessment of potential behavioural, social, communicative and environmental factors, to allow a diagnostic conclusion to be reached.

- **What would be your first choice of medication and why?**
  Maladaptive behaviour should always be managed using a behavioural approach. If however the response to behavioural measures is not sustained/ only partial and the behaviour is high risk, then medication may have to be considered alongside behavioural measures as a last resort. The treatment of aggression is dealt with in Chapter 12. Drug treatment of SIB should follow Mace and Mauk's model (Table 13.3).

Anxiety

Margaret, a 32-year-old woman with moderate to severe ID, living with her family, presented to services with a recent increase in agitation and SIB. Due to the level of irritability and agitation, she had been excluded from attending day centre activities. She was also reporting headaches and backache. Carers reported she was continuing to be unusually restless and was unable to focus on activities.

- **What is your differential diagnosis?**
 (i) Physical health causations, including hyperthyroidism, infection, migraine, PMS, etc.; also, more sinister pathologies may need to be ruled out, for example, brain tumour with bone secondaries.
 (ii) Mental health causations including depression, bipolar affective disorder and anxiety disorder.
(iii) Social/environmental issues, for example, changes at the day centre causing increased anxiety.
(iv) Communication difficulties.

(v) Exacerbation of symptoms of an underlying developmental disorder, for example, ASD and ADHD, can be secondary to any of the above or occur independently.

- **What investigations are indicated?**
Physical health review, including appropriate blood testing, and neuroimaging if appropriately given the history and presentation
Psychiatric review for mental health and developmental disorders and social, environmental and communication factors, with further assessment as indicated, for example, speech and language therapy assessment and behavioural observation

- **What support could Margaret be given to help her communicate her symptoms?**
Assessment by a Speech and Language Therapist and production of a communication passport will be important. Use of augmented communication strategies, for example, pictures and photos, can be put in place. Education for staff around how Margaret communicates and strategies to help both her understanding and use of communication may be needed.

- **What is the role of medication if Margaret is experiencing anxiety symptoms?**
Medication should only be required if Margaret's level of arousal is too high for her to engage in psychological therapies. Treatment options include SSRIs, benzodiazepines, buspirone and propranolol, and treatment choice should be tailored to Margaret's symptom profile, for example, propranolol for primarily physical anxiety symptoms. The principle of drug treatment is to use for 4–6 weeks then taper off; this allows time for the person's arousal level to reduce sufficiently to engage in psychological treatments.

Depression

Beatrice, a 55-year-old lady with moderate ID and epilepsy who usually resides in the family home, is seen at the day centre facility for routine 6-month follow-up of her epilepsy by the ID psychiatry team. She takes sodium valproate and her seizures are well controlled. Her key worker reports that, for the last 3 months, Beatrice has been displaying increasing restlessness, irritability and anger at times during her day activities, which is unlike her. She has been staying in a temporary respite facility for the last 6 weeks and has been coming in somewhat unkempt and smelling of body odour for the last 3 weeks. On talking to respite facility staff, it becomes apparent that Beatrice has been unwilling to accept personal care, screaming and appearing agitated when asked to take a bath. The staff have been reluctant to push the issue, as they report that Beatrice's father passed away from a heart attack four months ago while taking a bath and was found later by Beatrice and her mum.

On questioning, Beatrice is eating and sleeping as normal and continuing to get ready in the mornings to attend her day activities as usual.

Questions

• **What is your differential diagnosis?**

It is likely that Beatrice is experiencing a bereavement reaction to the death of her father, and her understanding of what has happened and the plan for her future needs to be explored. Equally, this could represent a depressive episode, possibly severe with psychotic features. Although appetite and sleep are normal, this may be due to concomitant sodium valproate treatment, which has modified the presentation of depression. Beatrice may be continuing to attend day centre because it forms part of her regular routine, and questioning as to her enjoyment/level of engagement with the activities and staff/other service users will be important, to highlight changes in interest and evidence of social withdrawal. Either way, the loss of her father has been compounded by other losses: the move out of the family home and the separation from her mum as well as her dad. It is possible that Beatrice could be experiencing the early stages of dementia, and removing her from her familiar environment and support structure will highlight such difficulties. A further possibility is PTSD, triggered by finding her father after his death, and this could explain her reluctance to bathe. A further consideration is any social, communication or environmental issues related to her placement at the respite facility. Adjusting to the new setting may be challenging for Beatrice, especially if she has ASD or traits in addition to her ID and epilepsy. The staff at the new setting may be struggling to communicate with her and their understanding and handling of her needs to be explored, in particular any signs or symptoms suggestive of abuse. It is also important to look at the impact of Beatrice's epilepsy and its treatment, including her compliance with medication and any evidence of breakthrough seizure activity, along with considering any potential underlying physical conditions such as anaemia and hypothyroidism, which may need treatment.

• **What management strategies could be tried if Beatrice has depression?**

Appropriately adapted CBT should be considered in the first instance; however, if this is insufficient or Beatrice is unable to engage, then drug treatment, with an SSRI in the first instance, should be considered.

• **What is the potential impact of drug treatment for depression on Beatrice's epilepsy, and how should this be managed?**

Caution should be used when commencing drug treatment, because of the potential for impact on seizure threshold. Advice can be sought from texts such as the Maudsley guideline on appropriate drug choice; however, general principles are start low and go slow, and make sure carers are aware of the potential risks and what to do if concerns arise.

Bipolar

Fatima is a 33-year-old lady with a diagnosis of moderate ID and challenging behaviour. Carers report a number of triggers for her behaviour including menstruation, physical ill health (particularly recurrent urine infections) and changes in the family home. She has been treated with risperidone for the past 5 years with initial benefit; however, her carers now feel this has become ineffective. At your request, carers keep a detailed behaviour record for several months and bring this to the next appointment. The record highlights episodes of agitation, restlessness, irritability, reduced sleep and appetite, associated with self-injury and aggression. The record highlights some relationship with the reported triggers; however, other episodes have no clear trigger.

- **What are the diagnostic possibilities?**

  Consideration of an underlying ASD is important here: the person's normal anxiety levels may be pushed to an intolerable degree by the additional factors described earlier. Looking at mental health causations, the most likely explanation is a mood disorder, and the challenge is then to tease out whether it is a unipolar depression or a bipolar affective disorder and, if the latter, whether it is rapid cycling. Careful charting of symptoms is essential to bring out any pattern present. It would also be useful to get corroborative reports and information from other settings, for example, day services, to highlight the impact of any environmental factors and look at consistency of symptoms across settings. A series of observations by a community nurse may also be required, for the same reasons.

  Other possibilities should also be considered, for example, a thorough physical workup of her existing physical complaints and an investigation for other relevant physical causations, for example, diabetes mellitus, is indicated: worries about non-co-operation with investigations and treatment, diagnostic overshadowing and value judgements about quality of life can still conspire to prevent a person with ID accessing the same resources as the general population.

- **What are the treatment options?**

  Management will be condition specific. With respect to choices for bipolar affective disorder, a mood stabiliser will be first line (Algorithm 16.1). Treatment of a rapid cycling mood disorder – something perhaps more commonly seen in ID than in the general population – can prove particularly challenging and often requires the use of two drugs (Algorithm 16.3).

- **What factors might influence the choice of mood stabiliser in this lady?**

  Drug choice will not only depend on efficacy, but on the patient's health issues and ability to cooperate with investigations. Lithium would often be chosen first line; however, in this case, it was deemed inappropriate due to poor compliance with investigations and the history of recurrent urine infections (lithium is excreted through the kidneys), and sodium valproate was chosen instead, with good response.

Schizophrenia

Charles is a 25-year-old man with mild ID. He has lived in a residential home for the past 7 years. Normally, he is a pleasant person who can travel independently. He has a stammer but can otherwise communicate reasonably.

Recently, he started to be irritable with staff and withdrawn and his smoking considerably increased. A few days later, he started sitting in the lounge through the night, watching movies and turning up the volume. He subsequently became physically aggressive and appeared to be talking to an unseen stimulus, when observed by staff. There is a history of some 'mental health problems' in his mother. In the past, Charles has 'got in with the wrong crowd' and used cannabis but denies current use. He is referred by the GP to ID psychiatry services for further assessment.

Questions

1 What are the diagnostic possibilities?

After ruling out physical health problems and environmental issues, diagnostic possibilities include:

A Drug-induced psychosis – Good history and test for drugs, look for association between drug use and onset of symptoms, collateral information from carers is important.

B Paranoid schizophrenia – Obtain information from the mother and check her mental health. Thorough history looking at psychotic symptoms, that is, auditory/visual hallucinations, persecutory delusions, delusions of thought interference and control and any passivity phenomena.

C Depressive episode with psychotic symptoms – Check for life events or change in the environment and family history of depression or any mental health problems and whether psychotic symptoms are mood congruent.

D Hypomanic episode – Look for previous history of mood disorder and any current treatment with antidepressants that can contribute to elevated mood, elated mood and disinhibited behaviour with mood congruent psychotic symptoms.

2 What would be the treatment options in terms of medication?

If a diagnosis of psychosis is confirmed, then it would be appropriate to initiate an atypical antipsychotic medication after having a discussion with patient and carers regarding side effects and reasons for using the medication. It is important that baseline blood tests and ECG are carried out prior to initiation of the medication. BMI and waist circumference need to be recorded at baseline, 6 months and annually as part of the metabolic monitoring. If compliance is an issue, then there has to be consideration to use of depot medication.

3 What other management strategies could be used?

Psychosocial aspects of management would include:

A Education of patient and carers about illness and need for therapy

B Improving awareness around the dangers of using illicit drugs and their effects on mental health

C Compliance therapy

D Assessment of available social support and provision of further support where required

E Recognition of early warning signs of psychosis with a good contingency plan to manage relapses

F Improving awareness of short- and long-term side effects of antipsychotic medications

Alcohol

A 56-year-old lady with mild LD is brought to the attention of the local ID services by her adult son. She has been drinking heavily for many years and despite multiple inpatient detoxes has never remained abstinent for more than a few months or fully engaged in treatment. She has experienced withdrawal seizures in the past and has also been admitted to hospital following head injuries sustained in domestic violence on many occasions. She has always said she wants to continue to drink. Her son reports a gradual increase in forgetfulness and deterioration in her self-care and care of her house. She has also lost weight.

- **What are the diagnostic possibilities?**
  Wernicke Korsakoff's psychosis, amnestic syndrome, unspecified dementia, dementia due to use of alcohol, depression, delirium and intracranial bleed (e.g. subdural haematoma). Other underlying physical illness such as liver failure, infection (e.g. TB) or neoplasm or anaemia.
- **What management strategies could be tried?**
  Consider admission and detoxification. Start vitamins. Full physical examination (including neurological and for signs of liver failure) with blood workup, ECG and CT scan head. Mental state assessment including cognitive and memory assessment. Referral for neuropsychiatry and occupational therapy workups. Management will depend on diagnosis, but she may need more support with activities of daily living and cognitive strategies to help her with her memory deficits and tasks of daily living. Assess her capacity to make decisions about continuing drinking and where she is living. Removing her from the environment in which she drinks and peer group with which she drinks will help her towards abstinence. If this is not possible, consider a wet hostel.
- **What is the role of medication in this case?**
  She is at risk of Wernicke's and is a dependent drinker so she should be given a multivitamin such as Pabrinex high potency for 3–5 days IM followed by oral thiamine and vitamin B. If she develops Wernicke's, she should be transferred to a medical ward and given IV Pabrinex. If she experiences a withdrawal seizure, then she should be given PD diazepam. If seizures persist, consider referral to a specialist for advice restarting antiepileptics. She is unlikely to benefit from medication for alcohol relapse prevention (acamprosate as she is not motivated, disulfiram would be risky as she is likely not to have capacity and she may consume alcohol without realising the effects, and naltrexone is only of short-term benefit). If she is depressed, try psychological and social strategies first as all antidepressants are metabolised through the liver. If she does need an antidepressant, prescribe low doses, monitor LFTs and discuss with mental health pharmacist.

Personality disorder

James is a 26-year-old Caucasian male with a mild level of ID. His problems started from late childhood; although ADHD was queried, a definitive diagnosis was not made. As a young adult, his behavioural problems included severe aggression towards people and property. He had very poor frustration tolerance, would act out without thinking, blame others for his actions, abuse alcohol and illicit medications and steal or indulge in similar antisocial behaviours. He had a number of girlfriends, often people who were less able than him, and he was prone to be violent towards them after arguments. He would report hearing voices at times when he was stressed. These would last for up to a week or 2 weeks during which time he would be very disturbed and neglecting his personal care.

- **What is the differential diagnosis?** Possibilities include antisocial personality disorder, borderline personality disorder, ADHD, depression and psychosis (possibly stress and/or drug induced).
- **Which symptoms should initially be targeted for treatment?** Aggression should be prioritised, given the high-risk nature of this behaviour. Alcohol and substance misuse should be tackled second, given their impact on impulse control and potential for long-term harm to James' mental and physical health.
- **What is your medication group of choice?** Drug choice for treatment of James' aggression will depend on the aetiology of this behaviour (e.g. affective aggression vs. predatory aggression; see Algorithm 19.1). Treatment of psychotic symptoms (Chapter 17) and alcohol/substance use (Chapter 18) will be according to the relevant condition/chapter.
- **How should drug medication be titrated to best manage James' condition?**
  Medication should only be used in combination with other strategies such as anger management, input from Drug and Alcohol Services.

  Principles of medication use are go low and slow and introduce and build up to the optimum dose of one medication at a time. Assessing compliance with treatment is important, for example, ensuring medication is taken supervised and random urine checks for evidence of ongoing substance use.

Reference

Bargiota A, Diamanti-Kandarakis E (2012) The effects of old, new and emerging medicines on metabolic aberrations in PCOS. *Therapeutic Advances in Endocrinology and Metabolism* 3(1): 27–47.

Summary of Syndromes Mentioned in the Guidelines

The Frith Prescribing Guidelines for People with Intellectual Disability, Third Edition.
Edited by Sabyasachi Bhaumik, David Branford, Mary Barrett and Satheesh Kumar Gangadharan.
© 2015 John Wiley & Sons, Ltd. Published 2015 by John Wiley & Sons, Ltd.

Syndrome	Incidence	Aetiology/genetics	Severity ID	Main features
Aicardi syndrome	200 cases by 1997	X-linked dominant	Severe	Agenesis of corpus callosum, severe visual defects (chorioretinal lacunae), infantile spasms with associated abnormal EEG (hypsarrhythmia), skeletal abnormalities especially of the ribs and spine. Usually presents in infants Progressive course with psychomotor slowing, kyphoscoliosis, visual failure and typically death by early adulthood
Angelman syndrome	1:15000	Absence of maternal 15q11-13	Severe	Neurogenetic disorder characterised by severe intellectual and developmental disability including speech delay, sleep disturbance, seizures, jerky movements (especially hand flapping). frequent laughter or smiling and usually a happy demeanour
Cornelia de Lange syndrome	1:40000–1:100000	Uncertain: most sporadic cases	Moderate/ severe	Typical facies (upturned nose, anteverted nostrils, arched eyebrows, long eyelashes, crescent-shaped mouth, long philtrum, high palate, micrognathia), limb abnormalities, failure to thrive due to gastro-oesophageal reflux (may lead to aspiration pneumonia and death). Autistic-like behaviours especially stereotypies. Limited speech: a few words. Small stature, self-injury, undescended testicles, eye abnormalities
Down syndrome	1:600	Trisomy 21	Mild/ moderate	Typical facies (upward outward slanting eyes, prominent epicanthic folds, wide nasal bridge), short stature, hyperreflexia, gastrointestinal and congenital heart abnormalities. Hypotonia in childhood becomes less marked with age. Failure to thrive in infancy replaced by predisposition to obesity after age 3. Hearing impairments common. Language/speech deficits independent of ID level. Alzheimer's changes after age 35
Fragile X syndrome	1:1000–1:2600 males	Distal arm Xq27.3 associated with FMR-1 gene	Mild/ moderate	Absence of FMR protein delays neuronal development. Females show less severe ID than males, milder phenotypic features and slower deterioration. Typical facies (macrocephaly, long face, large prominent ears). Connective tissue disorder may contribute to heart defects and infections. Autistic-like behaviours, socially anxious, disturbed by a variety of stressors and environmental changes
Lennox–Gastaut syndrome	1:1000000	Uncertain	Moderate/ severe	More common in males. Combination of generalised seizures (atypical absences, tonic seizures, atonic attacks, myoclonic seizures); inter-ictal EEG shows diffuse slow (2–3 Hz) spike-and-wave changes with bursts of fast activity (10 Hz) during sleep; slow mental development, often progressive ID

Syndrome	Prevalence	Genetics	ID severity	Clinical features
Lesch–Nyhan syndrome	1:380 000	X-linked recessive	Mild/moderate	Inborn error of purine metabolism results in raised uric acid; untreated results in severe aggression, self-injury and gout. The risk of profound ID and self-injury relates to the degree of enzyme deficiency. Also severe motor disability, dystonia, growth retardation, visual impairments, feeding problems, involuntary movements, hypotonia and seizures. Early death from renal or respiratory failure or infection
Phenylketonuria (PKU)	1:5000–1:14 000	Autosomal recessive	Moderate/severe	Absence of phenylalanine hydroxylase causes inability to metabolise phenylalanine. A phenylalanine-free diet from the first few weeks prevents ID. Inadequate dietary control may result in agitation, restlessness, intention tremor and tics. Neuropsychiatric symptoms arise if untreated
Prader–Willi syndrome	1:10 000	Abnormal paternal 15q11-13 in 60–70%	Borderline/moderate	Marked hypotonia, failure to thrive, delayed sexual development, scoliosis, small stature, persistent skin picking. Typical facies: prominent forehead with bitemporal narrowing, almond-shaped eyes, triangular mouth. Up to 6 months, hypotonia, feeding difficulties and sleepiness. Later hyperphagia arises from hypothalamic abnormalities. Psychiatric and behavioural problems increase with age
Rett syndrome	1:10 000 females	Distal arm of Xq28 75% MECP2 mutation	Profound	Diagnostic criteria: normal development until 6–18 months; deceleration of head growth; loss of verbal ability; stereotypic movements replace purposeful hand movements; failure to walk or abnormal gait; ataxic movements of torso/limbs, worse with distress. Regression of physical, social, linguistic and adaptive behaviours. Breathing abnormalities
Rubinstein–Taybi syndrome	1 in 125 000–300 000	Autosomal dominant or occurs de novo Mutations of CREBBP gene	Moderate/severe	Short stature, distinctive facial features, broad thumbs and first toes, cryptorchidism. Other features of the disorder vary among affected individuals. Additional features can include eye abnormalities, heart and kidney defects, dental problems and obesity. Increased risk of developing non-cancerous and cancerous tumours, leukaemia and lymphoma
Smith–Magenis syndrome	1:25 000	Partial/complete deletion of band 17p11.2	Moderate	Multiple congenital abnormalities, hearing/visual difficulties, scoliosis, sleep disturbance. Typical facies: brachycephaly, broad face and nasal bridge, flat midface, mouth turns down, cupid's bow shape upper lip, abnormal shape/position of ear. Self-injury, hyperactivity, aggression, need for 1:1 adult attention. Hypothyroidism, immunoglobulin deficiency, congenital heart disease

Syndrome	Incidence	Aetiology/genetics	Severity ID	Main features
Sturge–Weber syndrome	Unknown	Uncertain; cases sporadic	60% have ID of varying degree	Uncommon congenital disorder: unilateral/bilateral port-wine naevus (usually in distribution of trigeminal nerve), epilepsy, haemiparesis, mental impairment, eye problems (raised intraocular pressure, glaucoma/buphthalmos, field defects, choroidal naevi, colobomas of the iris). Seizures focal of generalised; mostly develop in the first year of life; brain damage following fits may worsen haemiplegia or mental impairment
Tuberous sclerosis	1:7000	Autosomal dominant 9q34.3 or 16p13.3	50% ID: severe/profound	Complex non-degenerative, neurocutaneous multi-system condition: diverse symptoms/severity. Sclerotic tuber-like growths may affect any part of the body; typically hamartias, hamartomas, neoplasia, facial angiofibromas. 50% have ID. 75% develop epilepsy. 50% autistic-like behaviour and/or hyperactivity (irrespective of level of ID). Cerebral and renal lesions having the highest mortality
West syndrome	Depends on cause	Various congenital brain malformations	Severe	Infantile spasms – flexor (salaam) and extensor myoclonic spasms of the neck, truck and links; hypsarrhythmic EEG; severe ID; onset < a year Common causes: Down syndrome, leucodystrophy, tuberous sclerosis, inborn errors of metabolism; prenatal infection; perinatal hypoxia
Williams syndrome	1:7500	Deletion of 7q11.23	Mild/moderate	A progressive multi-system syndrome with elfin facies; supravalvular aortic stenosis; ID with severe visuospatial/motor deficits; hyperacusis. Hypercalcaemia especially in infancy. Cardiovascular features, for example, hypertension, arterial stenosis, mitral valve collapse, kyphosis, scoliosis and joint contractures. Urinary and gastrointestinal problems, for example, constipation. Odd cognitive/personality profile with strong verbal ability relative to their IQ.

Index

The Frith Prescribing Guidelines for People with Intellectual Disability, Third Edition.
Edited by Sabyasachi Bhaumik, David Branford, Mary Barrett and Satheesh Kumar Gangadharan.
© 2015 John Wiley & Sons, Ltd. Published 2015 by John Wiley & Sons, Ltd.

Printed and bound by CPI Group (UK) Ltd, Croydon, CR0 4YY

27/10/2024

14580352-0001

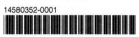